Hypertension Therapy Annual 2002

Hypertension Therapy Annual 2002

Edited by

Norman M Kaplan MD

Professor of Internal Medicine
University of Texas Southwestern Medical Center
Dallas, TX
USA

Martin Dunitz

© 2002 Martin Dunitz Ltd, a member of the Taylor & Francis group

First published in the United Kingdom in 2002 by
Martin Dunitz Ltd,
The Livery House,
7–9 Pratt Street, London NW1 0AE

Tel: +44 (0) 20 7482 2202
Fax: +44 (0) 20 7267 0159
E-mail: info@dunitz.co.uk
Website: http://www.dunitz.co.uk

A CIP record for this book is available from the British Library.

ISBN 1 84184 103 X

Although every effort has been made to ensure that all owners of copyright material have
been acknowledged in this publication, we would be glad to acknowledge in subsequent
reprints or editions any omissions brought to our attention.

Distributed in the USA by
Fulfilment Center
Taylor & Francis
7625 Empire Drive
Florence, KY 41042, USA
Toll Free Tel: +1 800 634 7064
E-mail: cserve@routledge_ny.com

Distributed in Canada by
Taylor & Francis
74 Rolark Drive
Scarborough, Ontario M1R 4G2, Canada
Toll Free Tel: +1 877 226 2237
E-mail:tal_fran@istar.ca

Distributed in the rest of the world by
ITPS Limited
Cheriton House
North Way
Andover, Hampshire SP10 5BE, UK
Tel: +44 (0)1264 332424
E-mail: reception@itps.co.uk

Composition by Wearset Ltd, Boldon, Tyne and Wear
Printed in Great Britain by Biddles Ltd, Guildford and King's Lynn

Contents

Contributors

Patrick Allen
Department of Therapeutics and Pharmacology, The Queen's University of Belfast, Northern Ireland.

George L Bakris
Rush University Hypertension Center, Department of Preventive Medicine, Rush Medical College, Chicago, IL, USA.

Chiara Bolego
Department of Medical Pharmacology, University of Milan, Italy.

Lennart Hansson
Clinical Hypertension Research, Department of Public Health and Social Sciences, University of Uppsala, Sweden.

Peter D Hart
Rush Medical College, and Hypertension Clinics, Cook County Hospital, Chicago, IL, USA.

Jiang He
Department of Epidemiology, School of Public Health and Tropical Medicine, Tulane University, New Orleans, Louisiana, USA.

Norman M Kaplan
University of Texas Southwestern Medical Center, Dallas, TX, USA.

Gary McVeigh
Department of Therapeutics and Pharmacology, The Queen's University of Belfast, Northern Ireland.

David Morgan
Department of Therapeutics and Pharmacology, The Queen's University of Belfast, Northern Ireland.

Paul Muntner
Department of Epidemiology, School of Public Health and Tropical Medicine, Tulane University, New Orleans, Louisiana, USA.

Rodolfo Paoletti
Department of Medical Pharmacology, University of Milan, Italy.

Andrea Poli
Department of Medical Pharmacology, University of Milan, Italy

Eberhard Ritz
Department of Internal Medicine, Ruperto Carola University, Heidelberg, Germany.

Michael Schömig
Department of Internal Medicine, Ruperto Carda University, Heidelberg, Germany.

†John D Swales
(Formerly) Leicester Royal Infirmary, Leicester, UK.

Paul Whelton
Department of Epidemiology, School of Public Health and Tropical Medicine, Tulane University, New Orleans, Louisiana, USA.

†deceased

Dedication

This book is dedicated to Professor John D Swales who died on 17 October 2000, at the age of 64. His contribution to the prior edition was only one of his many succinct, highly informative and usually provocative papers. Although I occasionally disagreed with his position, as on the question of the value of population-wide sodium reduction, I never doubted his sincerity, honesty and motivation in taking somewhat unpopular stances. He was a true gentleman, in the best sense of that word. Always considerate and thoughtful, he stood up forcefully for what he believed in.

His colleague, Bryan Williams, wrote an appropriate obituary, published in the February 2001 issue of the Journal of Hypertension – a journal for which John served as the first editor-in-chief. We are all thankful to have had John with us and we will miss him greatly.

1
Choice of initial therapy: new clinical trials data

Lennart Hansson

Introduction

Treatment of arterial hypertension is one of the therapeutic success stories of the twentieth century, comparable to the introduction of antibiotics in the combat of infectious diseases and the immunosuppressive drugs in transplantation medicine. It is the aim of this chapter to briefly discuss the choice of initial therapy for the treatment of hypertension: the pros and cons of the various classes of antihypertensive agents based on new clinical trial data will form the basis of this discussion. This task is facilitated by the fact that in the last few years several large intervention trials in hypertension have been completed and published. Some of these trials have compared active therapy to placebo and are perhaps of limited value in the context of choosing initial therapy, although some clinically useful information on drug selection can be extracted from such trials. Another group of intervention trials have evaluated two or more active antihypertensive therapies in head-to-head comparisons as regards their preventive effect against cardiovascular morbidity and mortality. Such trials, provided that they have been properly randomized, can obviously provide important information on the optimal choice of initial therapy.

A brief return to the early years of antihypertensive therapy, i.e. the 1950s and the early years of the 1960s, shows that the main emphasis was on the treatment of malignant hypertension, the most severe form of this disease. In its untreated form the 5-year survival was 0%, i.e. worse than most forms of cancer, but with the availability of antihypertensive drugs such as the ganglion blockers, reserpine and hydralazine 5-year survival was brought to 30–40% in a series of publications (*Table 1.1*).[1] All of these studies were uncontrolled and non-randomized but the positive message was so clear that the issue of producing confirmatory data from placebo-controlled and randomized trials was never raised. It is worth noting that many of these trials were conducted, and some even published, before diuretics became available in 1958.

In 1967 and 1970 the Veterans Administration (VA) study also showed

Table 1.1   Five-year survival in malignant hypertension

Authors	Number of patients	Year	Five-year survival (%)
Untreated			
Pickering et al.[6]	407	1961	0
Treated			
Dustan et al.[7]	84	1958	33
Harington et al.[8]	94	1959	22
Björk et al.[9]	93	1960	25
Sokolow and Perloff[10]	26	1960	15
Mohler and Freis[11]	64	1960	22
Hodge et al.[12]	497	1961	36
North et al.[13]	106	1961	44
Farmer et al.[14]	161	1963	29

Based on Hansson.[1]

convincing benefits of treatment in non-malignant hypertension.[2,3] The VA study was a randomized placebo-controlled trial of triple-drug treatment (reserpine + hydralazine + hydrochlorothiazide) in men with relatively severe hypertension (diastolic blood pressure 90–129 mmHg). The results of the VA study plus 12 other important intervention trials have been summarized in a well-known meta-analysis by Collins et al.[4] In brief, these trials showed that antihypertensive treatment based mainly, but not only, on diuretics or β-blockers conveyed useful reductions in cardiovascular morbidity attributable to a difference in diastolic blood pressure of only 5–6 mmHg when treated versus untreated or placebo patients.[4] That markedly better results can be achieved is shown when the results of the meta-analysis by Collins et al.[4] are compared with the results of the Hypertension Optimal Treatment (HOT) study in which the diastolic blood pressure was reduced by 20–24 mmHg, as compared to baseline, albeit not placebo corrected (*Table 1.2*).[5]

Table 1.2   Comparison of the HOT study[5] with the meta-analysis by Collins et al.[4]

	HOT[5]	Collins et al.[4]
Reduction in diastolic BP* (mmHg)	20–24	5–6
Patients achieving diastolic BP ≤90 mmHg (%)	92	55
Cardiovascular deaths per 1000 patient years	3.8	6.5
Myocardial infarctions per 1000 patient years	3.0	7.8

*BP, blood pressure.

The 13 trials included in the meta-analysis by Collins *et al.*[4] were taken to show that diuretics and/or β-blockers were useful in reducing cardiovascular morbidity in hypertensive patients, although it should be noted that in many of these trials substantial numbers of patients were given other antihypertensive agents as well. In fact, it would be fair to conclude that the main findings in these early and important trials were:

(a) the reduction in blood pressure *per se* is associated with reductions in cardiovascular morbidity and mortality;
(b) the positive results in this regard have, almost without exception, been obtained with combinations of antihypertensive drugs;
(c) no single class of antihypertensive agent was shown to be more effective in this regard than other classes;
(d) in studies where diuretics were an important component of the antihypertensive regimen, much higher doses – four- to eight-fold or more – were used as compared to current clinical practice.

Still, the usefulness of diuretics or β-blockers as first-line treatment for hypertension was confirmed in three large randomized and placebo-controlled trials in elderly hypertensive patients published in 1991 and 1992 (*Table 1.3*): the Systolic Hypertension in the Elderly Program (SHEP) study,[15] the Swedish Trial in Old Patients with Hypertension (STOP-Hypertension)[16] and the Medical Research Council (MRC) trial in older adults.

Taken together these 16 trials had an important impact on the treatment of hypertension and diuretics, and β-blockers were always amongst the drug classes recommended for first-line treatment in hypertension in various guidelines for the management of hypertension such as the various Joint National Committee (JNC) recommendations from the USA and those issued jointly by the World Health Organization and the International Society of Hypertension (WHO–ISH).

In recent years several important intervention trials in hypertension have been completed, assessing the effect of treatment on cardiovascular morbidity. Some have been comparisons between active therapy, usually a calcium antagonist, and placebo; others have been comparisons between two or more active therapies.

Most of the recent trials in the first category have used a calcium antagonist as active therapy, e.g. the Shanghai Trial Of Nifedipine in Elderly patients (STONE),[18] the Systolic Hypertension in Europe (Syst-Eur) study[19] and the Systolic Hypertension in China (Syst-China)[20] trials. Although much valuable information has been provided by these trials, they are obviously not ideally suited for the assessment of optimal initial therapy.

To this group could be added the Heart Outcomes Prevention Evaluation (HOPE) study, which also compared an active antihypertensive agent, the ACE inhibitor ramipril, with placebo.[21] It should be stressed

Table 1.3 Summary of the SHEP,[15] STOP-Hypertension[16] and MRC[17] intervention trials in elderly hypertensive patients

	SHEP[15]	STOP[16]	MRC[17]
Method	Double-blind	Double-blind	Single-blind
n	4736	1627	4396
Follow-up (years)	4.5	2.1	5.8
BP inclusion			
SBP* (mmHg)	160–219	180–230	160–209
DBP† (mmHg)	<90	>90	<115
Treatment	Chlorthalidone (+ atenolol)	Atenolol or metoprolol or pindolol or Moduretic	Atenolol or Moduretic
ΔBP (mmHg)	12/4	20/8	12/5
Results (% reduction)			
Deaths, all causes	13 (ns)	43 (p = 0.0079)	3 (ns)
Stroke, all	37 (p = 0.0003)	47 (p = 0.0081)	25 (p = 0.04)
CHD‡	25 (p < 0.05)	13 (MI)‖ (ns)	19 (ns)
CV§ events, all	32 (p < 0.01)	40 (p = 0.0031)	17 (p = 0.03)

*SBP, systolic blood pressure; †DBP, diastolic blood pressure; ‡CHD, coronary heart disease; §CV, cardiovascular; ‖MI, myocardial infarction.

that the HOPE study was not an intervention trial in hypertension, although some 60% of the patients in the diabetes substudy MICRO-HOPE were hypertensive.[22] Impressive reductions in cardiovascular risk were obtained in the high-risk patients recruited for the HOPE study by adding ramipril rather than placebo to whatever else these patients were taking.[21,22] However, since an active comparator was not used all one can say is that the angiotensin-converting-enzyme (ACE) inhibitor was significantly more effective than placebo in reducing risk.

The second group of recently completed intervention trials in hypertension consists of studies in which two or more active therapies have been compared as regards their effect on cardiovascular morbidity. Amongst these studies are the Captopril Prevention Project (CAPPP),[23] the Swedish Trial in Old Patients with Hypertension-2 (STOP-Hypertension-2),[24] the Nordic Diltiazem (NORDIL) study,[25] the International Nifedipine once-daily Study Intervention as a Goal in Hypertension Treatment (INSIGHT) study[26] and the United Kingdom Prospective Diabetes Study (UKPDS).[27] This group of trials is ideally suited for the assessment of the optimal choice of initial antihypertensive treatment, since patients were randomized to one of two or more active *initial* therapies. The reason is that all these studies have used combined treatment in substantial numbers of the enrolled patients in order to reach predetermined target blood pressure. This is not to say that combined therapy is a negative feature. On the contrary, in clinical practice this is how hypertension is managed. It is becoming increasingly clear that a majority of patients will need combinations of two or more antihypertensive drugs in order to lower blood pressure down to acceptable levels, a fact clearly illustrated in the HOT study, in which about two-thirds of all patients required combined treatment in order to reach their randomized blood pressure target (*Fig. 1.1*).[5]

A third large group of similar trials, i.e. comparing two or more active therapies, is still in progress and can obviously not yet contribute any information regarding the best choice of initial therapy. Those trials will not be dealt with here.

Recent intervention trials comparing placebo and active treatment

Shanghai Trial Of Nifedipine in Elderly patients (STONE) study

The STONE study, conducted in elderly patients in Shanghai, showed a statistically significant effect of nifedipine in reducing stroke.[18] Placebo or nifedipine was allocated in an alternate fashion, i.e. to every second patient. Thus, a proper randomization procedure was not used, detracting from the value of this trial.

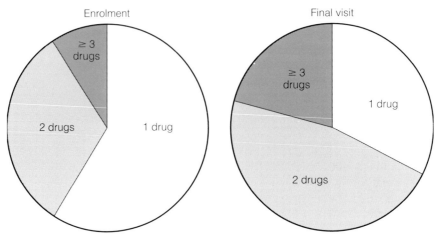

Figure 1.1

Combined antihypertensive treatment at baseline and at 3 years in the Hypertension Optimal Treatment (HOT) study in patients who were taking treatment when entering the study. Note the marked increase in the number of drugs and the associated markedly better control of blood pressure. Based on Hansson *et al.*[5]

Systolic Hypertension in Europe (Syst-Eur) study

This was the first intervention trial with appropriate randomization to show that a calcium antagonist-based antihypertensive regimen provides protection against cardiovascular morbidity.[19] The results affected the American JNC VI guidelines of 1997 which, based on the Syst-Eur study, listed long-acting dihydropyridine-derived calcium antagonists as being suitable for first-line treatment of elderly patients with isolated systolic hypertension.[28] A substantial proportion of patients received combined treatment with enalapril in the actively treated group.[19]

In a subgroup of patients with isolated systolic hypertension plus type 2 diabetes mellitus, at baseline, active antihypertensive treatment was equally effective in relative terms as in the whole study population.[29] These positive results confirmed the benefits of treating diabetic patients with isolated systolic hypertension, as already reported in a substudy of the SHEP study.[30]

Another interesting subgroup analysis showed that active antihypertensive treatment reduced the incidence of dementia, mainly Alzheimer's disease, by about 50%, $p = 0.05$.[31] This interesting aspect of antihypertensive therapy was already under investigation in the ongoing Study on Cognition and Prognosis in the Elderly (SCOPE), which is specifically assessing cognitive function in elderly hypertensives given either the AT$_1$-receptor antagonist candesartan cilexetil or placebo.[32] The SCOPE study is being conducted in several European countries, plus the USA and

Israel, and has recruited almost 5000 patients between the ages of 70 and 89. It is expected that the results will be available in 2002.

Systolic Hypertension in China (Syst-China) study

The Syst-China study[20] was a parallel study to the Syst-Eur trial.[19] Conducted in China it used the same inclusion criteria as the Syst-Eur study. The calcium antagonist-based treatment (nitrendipine + captopril if needed) significantly reduced all cardiovascular end-points (by 37%), stroke (by 38%) and all cardiac end-points (by 37%). As in the STONE study,[9] every second patient was allocated to placebo or active treatment, thus a regular randomization process was not used.

The results were very similar to those of the Syst-Eur trial. In other words, there are now two large intervention trials that demonstrate the benefits of calcium antagonist-based antihypertensive therapy in terms of reducing 'hard end-points' in patients with isolated systolic hypertension.

Recent intervention trials in which two or more active therapies were compared

As alluded to above, these trials are well suited to assess the choice of initial therapy in the treatment of hypertension. It should be noted that combined treatment has frequently been deemed necessary to reach the target blood pressure in all these trials. Almost without exception, the chosen first-step combinations have been between one 'new' and one 'old' drug, or, to use the JNC V nomenclature, between a 'preferred' and an 'alternative' drug.[33] In other words, the combinations have been between, for example, an ACE inhibitor and a diuretic or a calcium antagonist and a β-blocker. This means that the debate of whether to use the old and supposedly cheaper drugs rather than the new and supposedly more expensive drugs is now of limited interest. In this context it should also be pointed out that the total cost for treatment with preferred or alternative drugs is very similar (*Table 1.4*).[34]

Table 1.4   Costs for charging of preferred and alternative antihypertensive therapy*

Charges from	Preferred therapy[†]	Alternative therapy[‡]	p
Hospital/emergency room	323 ± 98	278 ± 186	ns
Clinic visits	354 ± 17	264 ± 29	0.005
Laboratory	336 ± 29	204 ± 56	0.010
Medications	319 ± 28	289 ± 38	ns

*Costs in US dollars: mean values ± standard derivation; †preferred therapy, β-blockers and diuretics; ‡alternative therapy, mainly ACE inhibitors and calcium antagonists († and ‡ according to JNC V).[33] Based on Elliot.[34]

Captopril Prevention Project (CAPPP) study

The CAPPP study was the first proper intervention trial in hypertension that compared outcome of treatment based on an ACE inhibitor with conventional treatment based on diuretics or β-blockers.[23] Obviously, ACE inhibitors had been widely used in the treatment of high blood pressure for many years before the CAPPP study was started. This class of agents had also been listed as first-line therapy for hypertension in several national and international guidelines, e.g. WHO–ISH in 1989.[35] Yet there existed no randomized intervention trial data with ACE inhibitors in hypertension to show that such treatment reduces cardiovascular morbidity or mortality.

In the CAPPP study, 11,018 hypertensive patients were studied in a prospective, randomized, open, blinded-end-point evaluation (PROBE) trial,[36] conducted at 475 health centres in Sweden and Finland. Patients between the ages of 25 and 66 with a diastolic blood pressure ≥100 mmHg on three occasions were randomized to receive either captopril or conventional (diuretics or β-blockers) antihypertensive treatment for an average of 5 years.

All primary cardiovascular events (fatal and non-fatal myocardial infarction and stroke, plus other cardiovascular mortality) were not different in the two groups, with a relative risk (RR) = 1.03 (ns) (*Fig. 1.2*).[23]

Cardiovascular mortality was lower in the captopril group, RR = 0.73, $p = 0.040$. Total mortality was numerically lower in the captopril group, but the difference was not statistically different, RR = 0.92 (ns).

There was a higher risk of suffering a stroke in the captopril group which was statistically significant. This could be explained by a more rapid and greater lowering of blood pressure in the group receiving conventional therapy. When comparing the results in the 5500 patients who

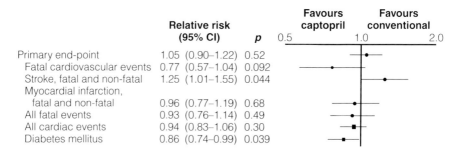

Figure 1.2

Relative risk (RR) of primary cardiovascular events (fatal and non-fatal myocardial infarction and stroke plus other cardiovascular mortality) in the Captopril Primary Prevention Project (CAPPP). From Hansson *et al.*[23] (published with permission).

were previously untreated, and in whom blood pressure fell to the same extent and at similar times in the two groups, there was no difference in the incidence of stroke. Thus, it was concluded that the ACE inhibitor-based regimen was not less protective against stroke than the conventional treatment.

The number of new cases of diabetes mellitus was significantly lower in the captopril group, a result which obviously has long-term prognostic implications.

Swedish Trial in Old Patients with Hypertension-2 (STOP-Hypertension-2) study

The STOP-Hypertension study[16] demonstrated reductions in stroke morbidity and mortality (47%), all cardiovascular end-points (40%) and in total mortality (43%) that were statistically significant when elderly hypertensives (70–84 years of age) were treated with a regimen that usually consisted of the combined use of a diuretic (Moduretic) and a β-blocker in a placebo-controlled trial.[16]

The STOP-Hypertension-2 study[24] was initiated following the positive results of the first STOP-Hypertension study.[16] It included 6614 patients, also 70–84 years of age.[24] The patients were randomized to one of three therapeutic arms:

(a) a diuretic/β-blocker arm using exactly the same drugs as in the STOP-Hypertension study, i.e. either of the β-blockers atenolol, metoprolol or pindolol, or hydrochlorothiazide + amiloride (Moduretic);[16]
(b) a calcium antagonist arm using felodipine or isradipine;
(c) an ACE inhibitor arm using enalapril or lisinopril.

The statistical calculations were based on the aim of demonstrating a 25% difference in cardiovascular mortality between the old and new therapies ($2p < 0.05$, with a power of 90%). The STOP-Hypertension-2 study was conducted in accordance with the PROBE design.[36]

The three therapeutic regimes were virtually identical in their blood pressure-lowering effect (*Table 1.5*).

Fatal cardiovascular events, i.e. the primary end-point, occurred in 221 patients in the group treated with conventional therapy (19.8 per 1000 patient–years) and in 438 patients in the group treated with newer agents (19.8 per 1000 patient–years); RR = 0.99 [95% confidence interval (CI) 0.84–1.16, $p = 0.89$].

Of the 438 fatal cardiovascular events, 226 occurred in patients on ACE inhibitors (20.5 per 1000 patient–years) and in 212 patients on calcium antagonists (19.2 per 1000 patient–years); the RR in comparison with conventional therapy were 1.01 (95% CI 0.84–1.22, $p = 0.89$) and 0.97 (95% CI 0.80–1.17, $p = 0.72$), respectively. RR in the ACE inhibitor group, when compared with the calcium antagonist group, was 1.04

Table 1.5   Supine blood pressure (mmHg) in the STOP-Hypertension-2 study

	Conventional	ACE inhibitors	Calcium antagonists
Randomization	194/98	194/98	194/98
1 month	173/88	174/89	172/88
6 months	165/85	167/86	167/85
12 months	165/85	167/86	167/85
24 months	163/84	164/84	165/84
36 months	161/83	163/83	163/82
48 months	161/82	162/82	162/82
54 months	158/81	159/81	159/80

From Hansson L et al.[24] (published with permission).

(95% CI 0.86–1.26, $p = 0.67$). Cardiovascular events in the three therapy groups are shown in *Figs. 1.3–1.6*.

The following comparisons between the two STOP-Hypertension studies[16,24] show the remarkable similarities in the two patient populations at the time of inclusion (the STOP-Hypertension-1 study mentioned first): average age 76 versus 76; recumbent systolic blood pressure 195 versus 194 mmHg; serum cholesterol 6.5 versus 6.5 µmol/l. For these reasons a comparison between the actively treated groups in the STOP-Hypertension-2 study[24] and the placebo group in the STOP-Hypertension study[16] was made. As expected, it showed that all the ther-

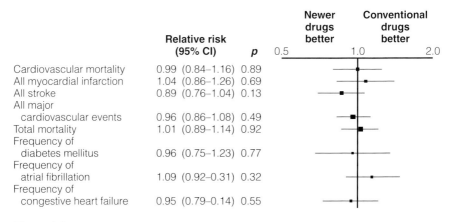

	Relative risk (95% CI)	p
Cardiovascular mortality	0.99 (0.84–1.16)	0.89
All myocardial infarction	1.04 (0.86–1.26)	0.69
All stroke	0.89 (0.76–1.04)	0.13
All major cardiovascular events	0.96 (0.86–1.08)	0.49
Total mortality	1.01 (0.89–1.14)	0.92
Frequency of diabetes mellitus	0.96 (0.75–1.23)	0.77
Frequency of atrial fibrillation	1.09 (0.92–0.31)	0.32
Frequency of congestive heart failure	0.95 (0.79–0.14)	0.55

Figure 1.3

Relative risk (RR) of cardiovascular mortality and morbidity for the newer drugs versus conventional drugs in the STOP-Hypertension-2 study. From Hansson et al.[24] (published with permission).

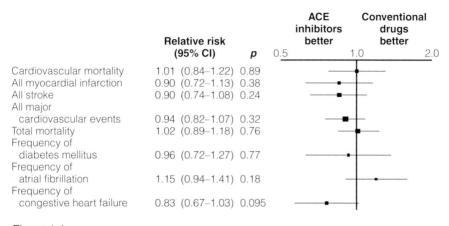

Figure 1.4
Relative risk (RR) of cardiovascular mortality and morbidity for the ACE inhibitors versus the conventional drugs in the STOP-Hypertension-2 study. From Hansson *et al.*[24] (published with permission).

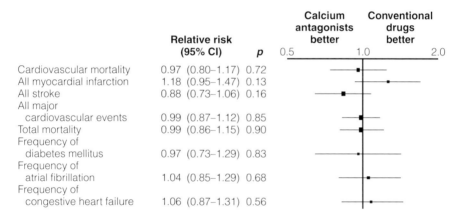

Figure 1.5
Relative risk (RR) of cardiovascular mortality and morbidity for the calcium antagonists versus conventional drugs in the STOP-Hypertension-2 study. From Hansson *et al.*[24] (published with permission).

apies used in the STOP-Hypertension-2 trial were more effective in preventing hard end-points than placebo.[24]

Nordic Diltiazem (NORDIL) study

The design of the NORDIL study[25] was very similar to that of the CAPPP study.[23] It was conducted at primary health-care centres in Sweden and

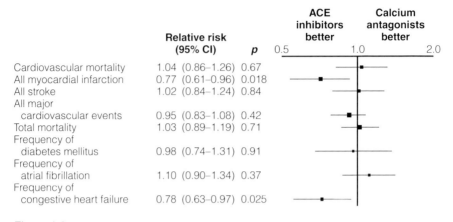

Figure 1.6

Relative risk (RR) of cardiovascular mortality and morbidity for the ACE inhibitors versus calcium antagonists in the STOP-Hypertension-2 study. From Hansson *et al.*[24] (published with permission).

Norway. This trial was the first intervention trial in hypertensive patients that compared the effect of a non-dihydropyridine calcium antagonist-based therapeutic regimen, using diltiazem, with that of a regimen based on diuretics and/or β-blockers, on cardiovascular morbidity and mortality.

In the NORDIL study, 10,881 hypertensive patients were studied in a PROBE trial.[36] Patients between the ages of 50 and 74 with a diastolic blood pressure ≥ 100 mmHg were randomized to receive antihypertensive treatment based on either diltiazem (Cardizem) or therapy based on diuretics and/or β-blockers for an average of 4.5 years.

Office blood pressure was lowered effectively in both groups, the reduction being 20.3/18.7 mmHg in the diltiazem-based group and 23.3/18.7 mmHg in the diuretics/β-blocker group.

The primary end-point of fatal and non-fatal stroke and myocardial infarction, plus other cardiovascular mortality, occurred in 403 patients in the diltiazem group (16.6 events per 1000 patient–years) and in 400 patients (16.2 events per 1000 patient–years) in the diuretic/β-blocker group; RR = 1.00 (95% CI 0.87–1.15, p = 0.97).

Fatal and non-fatal stroke occurred in 159 patients in the diltiazem group (6.4 events per 1000 patient–years) and in 196 patients (7.9 events per 1000 patient–years) in the diuretic/β-blocker group; RR = 0.80 (95% CI 0.65–0.99, p = 0.04). Fatal and non-fatal myocardial infarction occurred in 183 patients in the diltiazem group (7.4 events per 1000 patient–years) and in 157 patients (6.3 events per 1000 patient–years) in the conventional group; RR = 1.16 (95% CI 0.94–1.44, p = 0.17) (*Fig. 1.7*).

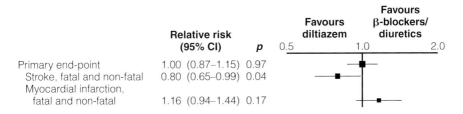

	Relative risk (95% CI)	p
Primary end-point	1.00 (0.87–1.15)	0.97
Stroke, fatal and non-fatal	0.80 (0.65–0.99)	0.04
Myocardial infarction, fatal and non-fatal	1.16 (0.94–1.44)	0.17

Figure 1.7

Relative risk (RR) of primary cardiovascular events (fatal and non-fatal myocardial infarction and stroke plus other cardiovascular mortality) in the Nordic Diltiazem Study (NORDIL). From Hansson et al.[25] (published with permission).

As regards all other studied end-points, i.e. cardiovascular death, fatal myocardial infarction, fatal stroke, all death, all cardiac events, transient ischaemic attacks, diabetes mellitus, atrial fibrillation and congestive heart failure, RR was between 1.16 and 0.82, none of which were statistically significant. In patients with type 2 diabetes mellitus, at baseline there were no significant differences in outcome between the two groups.

International Nifedipine once-daily Study Intervention as a Goal in Hypertension Treatment (INSIGHT) study

The INSIGHT study was a multinational (Europe and Israel) prospective double-blind trial in 6321 high-risk hypertensive patients between the ages of 55 and 80.[26] Patients were randomly assigned to treatment with either nifedipine 30 mg in long-acting gastrointestinal system (GITS) formulation or co-amilozide (hydrochlorothiazide 25 mg + amiloride 2.5 mg).

The effect on blood pressure was similar in the two groups and overall mean blood pressure fell from 173/99 to 138/82 mmHg.[26] There was an 8% excess withdrawal rate in the nifedipine group due to peripheral oedema (725 versus 518, $p < 0.0001$) but serious adverse events were more common in the diuretic group (880 versus 796, $p = 0.02$).

The two therapeutic modalities were equally effective in preventing cardiovascular complications (strokes plus myocardial infarctions plus congestive heart failure plus cardiovascular deaths), 18.2 versus 16.5 such events per 1000 patient–years in the two groups, respectively (RR = 1.10, $p = 0.35$).[26]

United Kingdom Prospective Diabetes Study (UKPDS)

The UKPDS was a trial in patients with type 2 diabetes mellitus conducted in the UK:[27] there were 1148 such patients who also had hypertension. The main emphasis in this important study was to compare 'tight' control of blood pressure (or blood sugar) with 'less tight' control.[18] However, in the present context, the comparison between captopril and atenolol in tight blood pressure control is of greater interest. In brief, there was no difference in outcome between these two therapies, although the ACE inhibitor regiment was better tolerated.[37] Although, it must be pointed out that the study was vastly underpowered to address this issue adequately.

Discussion

In several recent large hypertension intervention trials two or more active antihypertensive therapies have been compared as regards their effect on cardiovascular morbidity and mortality.[23–27] The fact that patients were randomized to active treatments makes it possible to assess the pros and cons of the initial active therapies. Perhaps unexpectedly, the trials that have been published so far have not been able to distinguish clear advantages or disadvantages with the therapeutic modalities that have been studied. Admittedly, some subgroup analyses have shown statistically significant differences, e.g. a better preventive effect against myocardial infarction with ACE inhibitors than with calcium antagonists in the STOP-Hypertension-2 study[24] or a better protection against stroke with cardizem than with diuretics and/or β-blockers in the NORDIL study.[25] However, such subgroup findings should be looked upon with some caution: they may be chance findings. In order to accumulate sufficient numbers of end-points, and thereby attain adequate statistical power, one must await the results of the ongoing prospective collaborative overviews of major randomized trials of blood pressure-lowering treatments conducted by the WHO–ISH collaboration.[38]

While awaiting this important analysis, based on 35 major intervention trials, some important clinical conclusions can be drawn:

(a) The lowering of blood pressure *per se* is of major importance, as clearly shown in high-risk patients, e.g. those with hypertension and type 2 diabetes mellitus, compare the HOT study diabetic subgroup (n = 1501)[5] and the UKPDS (n = 1148).[27] It is interesting to note that the well-being of patients actually increases the lower the level of blood pressure attained, as shown in a substudy of the HOT study.[39]

(b) The choice of initial therapy has so far not been shown to be of critical importance in the reduction of cardiovascular morbidity or mortality.

(c) It is conceivable that certain end-points, such as stroke or myocardial infarcts, may be more or less effectively prevented by different compounds. In order to achieve sufficient statistical power for reliable conclusions in this regard, meta-analyses of relevant data are needed. By selectively including or excluding trials in such analyses it is probably possible to demonstrate whatever the investigator sets out to show. It would therefore appear prudent to await the large ongoing collaborative meta-analysis that is in progress under the auspices of WHO–ISH.[38]

(d) The lack of a distinct 'ideal choice' drug for initial treatment of hypertension has the advantage that virtually all the major drug classes can be used as first-line treatment. As alluded to above, the fact that most patients will need combinations of two or more antihypertensive drugs to reach an adequate target blood pressure, and the fact that the overall costs are very similar for the different drug regimens,[34] means that the treatment of hypertension can be strictly individualized, as it should be. With today's many therapeutic alternatives for the treatment of hypertension it should be possible to find effective and well-tolerated regimens for virtually all patients.

References

1. Hansson L. The benefits of lowering elevated blood pressure: a critical review of studies of cardiovascular morbidity and mortality in hypertension. J Hypertens 1996; 14: 537–544.

2. Collins R, Peto R, MacMahon S et al. Blood pressure, stroke, and coronary heart disease. Part 2, short-term reductions in blood pressure: over-view of randomised drug trials in their epidemiological context. Lancet 1990; 335: 827–838.

3. Veterans Administration Cooperative Study Group on Antihypertensive Agents. Effects of treatment on morbidity in hypertension. Results in patients with diastolic blood pressure averaging 115 through 129 mmHg. JAMA 1967; 202: 1028–1034.

4. Veterans Administration Cooperative Study Group on Antihypertensive Agents. Effects of treatment on morbidity in hypertension. II. Results in patients with diastolic blood pressure averaging 90 through 114 mmHg. JAMA 1970; 213: 1143–1152.

5. Hansson L, Zanchetti A, Carruthers SG et al. for the HOT Study Group. Effects of intensive blood pressure lowering and low-dose aspirin in patients with hypertension. Principal results of the Hypertension Optimal Treatment (HOT) randomised trial. Lancet 1998; 351: 1755–1762.

6. Pickering GW, Cranston WI, Pears MA. The treatment of hypertension. Charles C Thomas: Springfield, 1961.

7. Dustan HP, Schneckloth RE, Corcoran AC, Page IH. The effectiveness of long-term treatment of malignant hypertension. Circulation 1958; 18: 644–651.

8. Harington M, Kincaid-Smith P, McMichael J. Results of treatment in malignant hypertension. A 7-year experience in 94 cases. BMJ 1959; 2: 969–980.

9. Björk S, Sannerstedt R, Falkheden T, Hood B. The effect of active drug treatment in severe hypertensive disease. An analysis of survival rates in 381 cases of combined treatment with various

hypotensive agents. Acta Med Scand 1960; 166: 175–187.

10. Sokolow M, Perloff D. Five years' survival of consecutive patients with malignant hypertension treated with antihypertensive agents. Am J Cardiol 1960; 6: 858–863.

11. Mohler ER Jr, Freis ED. Five years' survival of patients with malignant hypertension treated with anti-hypertensive agents. Am Heart J 1960; 60: 329–335.

12. Hodge JV, McQueen EG, Smirk H. Results of hypotensive therapy in arterial hypertension based on experience with 497 patients treated and 156 controls observed for periods from 1 to 8 years. BMJ 1961; 1: 1–7.

13. North JDK, Williams JCP, Howie RN. Severe hypertension treated with ganglion-blocking drugs in a general hospital. BMJ 1961; 1: 1426–1429.

14. Farmer RG, Gifford RW, Hines EA. Effect of medical treatment of severe hypertension. A follow-up of 161 patients with group 3 and group 4 hypertension. Arch Inter Med 1963; 112: 118–128.

15. SHEP Cooperative Research Group. Prevention of stroke by hypertensive drug therapy in older persons with isolated systolic hypertension: final results of the systolic hypertension in the elderly program. JAMA 1991; 265: 3255–3264.

16. Dahlöf B, Lindholm LH, Hansson L et al. Morbidity and mortality in the Swedish trial in Old Patients with Hypertension (STOP-Hypertension). Lancet 1991; 338: 1281–1285.

17. MRC Working Party. Medical Research Council trial of treatment of hypertension in older adults: principal results. BMJ 1992; 304: 405–412.

18. Gong L, Zhang W, Zhu Y, et al. and 11 collaborating centres in the Shanghai area. Shanghai trial of nifedipine in the elderly (STONE). J Hypertens 1996; 14: 1237–1245.

19. Staessen JA, Fagard R, Thijs L et al. for the Systolic Hypertension in Europe (Syst-Eur) Trial Investigators. Randomised double-blind comparison of placebo and active treatment for older patients with isolated systolic hypertension. Lancet 1997; 350: 757–764.

20. Liu L, Wang JG, Gong L et al. for the Systolic Hypertension in China (Syst-China) Collaborative Group. Comparison of active treatment and placebo for older Chinese patients with isolated systolic hypertension. J Hypertens 1998; 16: 1823–1829.

21. Heart Outcomes Prevention Evaluation Study Investigators. Effects of an angiotensin-converting-enzyme inhibitor, ramipril, on death from cardiovascular causes, myocardial infarction, and stroke in high risk patients. N Engl J Med 2000; 342: 145–153.

22. Heart Outcomes Prevention Evaluation (HOPE) Study Investigators. Effects of ramipril on cardiovascular and microvascular outcomes in people with diabetes mellitus: results of the HOPE study and the MICRO-Hope substudy. Lancet 2000; 355: 253–259.

23. Hansson L, Lindholm LH, Niskanen L et al. for the Captopril Prevention Project (CAPPP) Study Group. Effect of angiotensin-converting-enzyme inhibition compared with conventional therapy on cardiovascular morbidity and mortality in hypertension: the Captopril Prevention Project (CAPPP) randomised trial. Lancet 1999; 353: 611–616.

24. Hansson L, Lindholm LH, Ekbom T et al. for the STOP-Hypertension-2 study group. Randomised trial of old and new antihyperten-

sive drugs in elderly patients: cardiovascular mortality and morbidity the Swedish Trial in Old Patients with Hypertension-2 study. Lancet 1999; 354: 1751–1756.

25. Hansson L, Hedner T, Lund-Johansen P et al. for the NORDIL Study Group. Randomised trial of effects of calcium antagonists compared with diuretics and β-blockers on cardiovascular morbidity and mortality in hypertension: the Nordic Diltiazem (NORDIL) study. Lancet 2000; 356: 359–365.

26. Brown MJ, Palmer CR, Castaigne A et al. Morbidity and mortality in patients randomised to double-blind treatment with a long-acting calcium-channel blocker or diuretic in the International Nifedipine GITS study; Intervention as a goal in Hypertension Treatment (INSIGHT). Lancet 2000; 356: 366–372.

27. UK Prospective Diabetes Study Group. Tight blood pressure control and risk of macrovascular and microvascular complications in type 2 diabetes: UKPDS 38. BMJ 1998; 317: 703–713.

28. Joint National Committee on Prevention, Detection, Evaluation, and Treatment of High Blood Pressure. The sixth report of the Joint National Committee on Prevention, Detection, Evaluation, and Treatment of High Blood Pressure. Arch Intern Med 1997; 157: 2413–2446.

29. Tuomilehto J, Rastenyte D, Birkenhäger WH et al. for the Systolic Hypertension in Europe Trial Investigators. Effects of calcium-channel blockade in older patients with diabetes and systolic hypertension. N Engl J Med 1999; 340: 677–684.

30. Curd JD, Pressel SL, Cutler JA et al. for the Systolic Hypertension in the Elderly Program Cooperative Research Group. Effect of diuretic-based antihypertensive treatment on cardiovascular disease risk in older diabetic patients with isolated systolic hypertension. JAMA 1996; 276: 1886–1892.

31. Forette F, Seux M-L, Staessen JA et al. on behalf of the Syst-Eur Investigators. Prevention of dementia in randomised double-blind placebo-controlled Systolic Hypertension in Europe (Syst-Eur) trial. Lancet 1998; 352: 1347–1351.

32. Hansson L, Lithell H, Skoog I et al. for the SCOPE Investigators. Study on cognition and prognosis in the elderly (SCOPE). Blood Pressure 1999; 8: 177–183.

33. Joint National Committee on Detection, Evaluation, and Treatment of High Blood Pressure. The fifth report of the Joint National Committee on Detection, Evaluation, and Treatment of High Blood Pressure (JNC V). Arch Intern Med 1993; 153: 154–183.

34. Elliot WJ. Costs associated with changing antihypertensive drug monotherapy: 'preferred' vs. 'alternative' therapy (abstract). Am J Hypertens 1995; 8: 80A.

35. World Health Organization–International Society of Hypertension (WHO–ISH) Fifth Mild Hypertension Conference. The 1989 guidelines for the management of mild hypertension. Memorandum from a WHO–ISH meeting. J Hypertens 1989; 7: 689–693.

36. Hansson L, Hedner T, Dahlöf B. Prospective Randomized Open Blinded End-point (PROBE) Study: A novel design for intervention trials. Blood Press 1992; 1: 113–119.

37. UK Prospective Diabetes Study Group. Efficacy of atenolol and captopril in reducing risk of macrovascular and microvascular complications in type 2 diabetes: UKPDS 39. BMJ 1998; 317: 713–720.

38. World Health Organization – International Society of Hypertension Blood Pressure Lowering Treatment Trialists' Collaboration. Protocol for prospective collaborative overviews of major randomized trials of blood-pressure lowering treatments. J Hypertens 1998; 353: 611–616.

39. Wiklund I, Halling K, Rydén-Bergsten T, Fletcher A, on behalf of the HOT Study Group. Does lowering the blood pressure improve the mood? Quality-of-life results from the Hypertension Optimal Treatment (HOT) Study. Blood Press 1997; 6: 357–364.

2
Guidelines for evaluation and therapy of hypertension

†John D Swales

Introduction

In 1999 updated versions of three sets of influential guidelines for managing hypertension were published.[1-3] In addition, many national specialist societies in developed countries issue guidance to professionals in their geographical areas. These usually follow closely the recommendations of the World Health Organization–International Society of Hypertension (WHO–ISH) group or those of the Joint National Committee on Prevention, Detection, Evaluation and Treatment of High Blood Pressure (JNC VI).[4] In developing parts of the world such as sub-Saharan Africa, where the need for advice to meet local conditions is at its greatest, less has been done. A recent survey showed that only the Nigerian Hypertension Society had produced guidelines,[5] although earlier guidelines have also been developed for primary-care professionals in South Africa.[6] Guidelines produced for the developed world reflect socio-economic conditions which make them largely inapplicable to less affluent societies. It would seem extremely important that guidance appropriate to the realities of health-care delivery and public health is produced in such countries. Pilot studies in Tanzania and the Cameroons are encouraging.[7]

The way in which hypertension is prevented or managed is powerfully influenced by the social and cultural environment in which it takes place. This is evident even in the guidelines produced for developed societies, where guideline development for all fields of clinical medicine has become something of an industry and serious questions have been raised about the effectiveness and value of the operation.[8,9] Nevertheless, regular reviews of management by independent expert groups provides an excellent way of defining the areas of practice where there is general agreement. Differences, by contrast, reflect divergent interpretation of the available scientific evidence and genuine differences in the judgement of what is worthwhile. The distinction between the two is usually not made explicit.

This chapter will focus on five widely disseminated, English-language guidelines.[1-4,10] These provide an excellent resume of expert views of best practice. Others, such as those produced in Australia,[11] which closely follow the WHO–ISH model, will not be discussed in detail.

Target audience

The first question to be asked of any published guidelines is: to whom are they addressed? Many professionals are concerned about the use of recommendations intended for clinicians by others pursuing a quite different agenda. Such interested parties include lawyers, governments, and purchasers and managers of health care.[12] The dangers are that innovative care may be inhibited and the flexibility required in meeting individual patient needs and wishes constrained. In the face of such concerns, recommendations should specify their target audience. Although this is unlikely to prevent misuse, it will help to focus the attention of those who prepare recommendations on the needs of those whom they are intended to help. Misuse is more likely when guidelines are unnecessarily prescriptive or dangerously vague in meeting these needs.

All define their target but with significant differences. The WHO–ISH committee recognizes a diversity of audiences by specifying 'specialist physicians' in the main report but also issues a companion set of 'practice guidelines' for general practitioners.[1] The British Hypertension Society guidelines list 'general practitioners, practice nurses and generalists in hospital practice' but are published separately in full and abbreviated forms.[2,13] The Canadian recommendations address 'health-care professionals' but define their work slightly differently as 'a technical document for the development of both clinical practice guidelines and a broader implementation strategy'.[3] JNC VI is defined as providing guidance for 'primary-care physicians' but goes on to describe the report as a 'tool to be adopted and implemented in local and individual situations'. The New Zealand guidelines are also directed at general practitioners but are unique in being produced by a statutory body – the Core Services Committee – which also advises the New Zealand government on 'the services it thinks should be secured'.[10]

Overall approach

With the exception of the New Zealand committee, all groups have produced guidelines regularly since the 1980s. The evolution of these documents reflects two processes: (a) the generation of new evidence; (b) changes in approach to that evidence. Recommendations to treat progressively lower blood pressure levels in all groups of patients, a growth in emphasis upon hypertension in the elderly and systolic blood pressure, and the importance of lifestyle modifications, as well as pharmacological treatment, have all been the result of new trial data. On the other hand, there have been equally conspicuous changes that cannot be directly related to the accumulation of new evidence. All guidelines now recommend assessment of overall cardiovascular risk and most have moved toward a much more rigorous quantitative or semi-quantitative evaluation of risk based upon epidemiologic data following the pioneering New Zealand recommendations.

There is also a more structured approach to evidence. The earlier Canadian recommendations spearheaded an evidence-based approach in which supportive scientific evidence was strictly graded.[14] Systematic reviews of end-point trials are placed at the top of a hierarchy of evidence, while observational data, arguments from physiological processes and expert opinion are allocated a lower grading. While advocates of evidence-based medicine state categorically that all levels of evidence may have to be used,[15] the preference attached to outcome trials as a gold standard ignores, in the present author's view, the essentially integrative process of clinical decision making[16] and carries a danger of a mechanistic approach to recommendations. Few individual patients meet the criteria necessary for inclusion in end-point trials, as the JNC guidelines point out in what is basically a caveat about the evidence-based approach.[4] Clinical practice inevitably necessitates a degree of extrapolation, using observational and uncontrolled clinical data. The more rigid evidence-based method has important consequences for the advice given. The use of multiple risk-factor profiling and risk calculation as a guide to treatment is dependent upon observational data. The Canadian recommendations are alone in not using such an approach, although it would have been consistent with their recommendations elsewhere which use lower levels of evidence where outcome trials do not exist. The American guidelines compromise by classifying cited evidence according to its nature. The British guidelines also classify supportive evidence in summary boxes but without defining its source. Since even meta-analyses have produced divergent conclusions, this would seem irrational.

Guidelines and economic cost

Health care is a costly process and subject to severe pressures across the world. Therefore, recommendations can only be implemented at a cost. This presents any specialist body with a number of difficult quandaries. The Canadian recommendations are unique in stating at the outset that 'neither public health policy nor economic considerations' contributed to their report. Other guidelines refer briefly to the importance of considering cost, particularly in the context of drug selection, although none attempts to evaluate the overall cost of the recommendations they are making for patient management. Despite this, implicit concern with cost must have played some role in recommendations, even those made by the Canadian group. Benefits in the investigation and treatment of hypertension are graded and not dichotomous. To take a simple example, the detection of an aldosterone-secreting adenoma of the adrenal cortex is often beneficial where it is revealed by laboratory investigations. While all guidelines recommend measurement of serum electrolytes in newly diagnosed hypertension, this procedure in isolation will result in the diagnosis being missed in a proportion of patients whose serum potassium, even taken under the most rigorous conditions, is normal. Most of these patients will be detected by measurement of the plasma aldosterone/renin ratio followed by more intensive investigation.[17] In the face of a very low prevalence of normokalaemic hyperaldosteronism due to adenoma, most clinicians (and guidelines) would regard routine screening in this way as not being justified. If, on the other hand, the prevalence was much higher, as some groups have suggested,[17] the case would be a strong one. Exactly the same arguments apply to the recommendations for the treatment of patients at lower absolute risk. Such examples underline the fundamental impossibility of providing advice for patient management which do not in some unacknowledged way consider likely benefit in relation to cost.

This raises a second, fundamental, question. If the costs of treating such a common chronic condition are considerable, the costs of untreated hypertension are also very great. The JNC VI guidelines point out that 'hypertension-associated heart disease, stroke and renal failure . . . often lead to expensive hospitalizations, surgical procedures and high-cost technologies' and that the cost of these exceeds the cost of managing hypertension. The British guidelines are, at one point, the most explicit of all about cost but also seem to have overlooked the consequential costs of failure to treat when they append a note to their risk factor table stating that; 'As a minimum, those at highest risk (⩾30%) should be targeted and treated now, and as resources allow others with a risk of >15% should be progressively targeted'. The issue is an important one. Narrow focus upon the short-term consequences for drug or health-care budgets overlooks the impact of failure to treat on long-term complications. The burden of avoidable cerebrovascular disease falls, for instance, not simply on health-care provision but upon social care, as well as upon individual patients and their families. The overall cost to society of dealing with these far exceeds the cost of controlling blood pressure.[18] The professionals who compile guidelines necessarily focus on the consequences of their advice for the health-care system in which most of them work: likewise, governments who are encouraging the development of cost awareness in clinical guidelines have created water tight boundaries between different budgets. Attention tends to be focused on drug costs or professional time rather than on the overall balance between the costs of treating versus not treating for society. Clinicians are taught to consider the impact of what they advise on every dimension of their patient's life and it would seem important for professional guidance to take a similarly broad view.

The third concern relates to equity when resources are constrained. Specialist groups are not equipped to ensure that the levels of risk and benefit at which they target their recommended interventions are set at a comparable level with recommendations for other conditions. This is difficult to achieve even in closely related fields such as the treatment of hypertension and dyslipidaemia. Thus, while the British Hypertension guidelines recommend that treatment is targeted at patients with a 10-year risk of 15% for coronary heart disease, the guidelines in the same document for statin treatment of dyslipidaemia target a 10-year risk of 30%. The justification for the latter is economic – 'workload for general practitioners and the enormous potential cost'. The degree of comparability with guidelines for managing other conditions is impossible to assess. JNC VI in 1997, for instance, recommends rechecking blood pressure in normotensive subjects at 2-year intervals. The same year, an American Expert Committee on Diabetes recommended screening for those over 45 years of age every 3 years for diabetes.[19] Neither recommendation attempted to estimate the amount of avoidable cardiovascular disease that would be detected by adopting these different strategies and whether they were comparable. It is probably unreasonable to expect expert committees to take a wide-ranging view of medical treatment. In any case, patients attach different values to different potential net outcomes of treatment. Equity across different interventions is best devolved to the clinicians who manage their individual needs. This is easier to achieve so long as guidelines are treated as a broad framework: when they become more prescriptive in tone, it is inevitable that serious anomalies will arise.

Comparison of guidelines

It is reassuring that, despite differences in approach and socio-cultural background, there is general agreement about the principles for evaluating and treating hypertension (*Fig. 2.1*). Initial clinical evaluation and lifestyle advice is followed by early or immediate pharmacological treatment of patients at higher levels of absolute risk. The majority of patients are then observed for a period of time determined by their level of risk. At the end of this period, if their blood pressure or individual risk exceeds a threshold value, they are offered antihypertensive medication. If not, blood pressure is monitored at defined intervals. In either case, patients are encouraged to persevere with lifestyle modification.

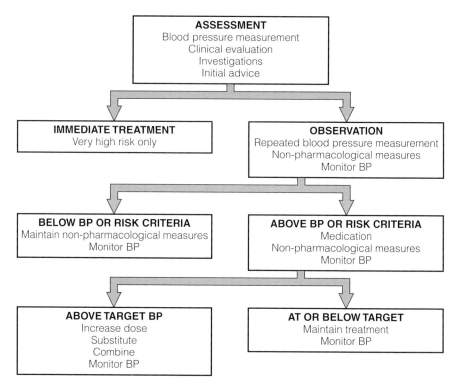

Figure 2.1

Treatment plan for hypertension. (BP, blood pressure.)

Evaluation

Patient management for any condition demands evaluation by means of history, examination and relevant laboratory tests and procedures. In the case of hypertension, there are several distinct objectives. These are:

(a) to evaluate the severity of hypertension;
(b) to detect the presence of contributory factors or, in the case of secondary hypertension, causes of high blood pressure;
(c) to assess overall cardiovascular risk from the presence of target-organ damage and other risk factors;
(d) to detect co-morbidity that may require treatment in its own right, or which may influence antihypertensive treatment.

All guidelines provide detailed recommendations for blood pressure assessment. There is a broad spectrum of advice on clinical history and examination, ranging from JNC VI and the WHO–ISH guidelines, that provide detailed listings of what should be sought, to the Canadian

Table 2.1   Recommended laboratory investigations in uncomplicated hypertension

Urinalysis
Blood cell count
Blood biochemistry
   potassium
   sodium
   creatinine
   fasting glucose
Blood lipids
   total cholesterol
   High-density lipoprotein cholesterol
Twelve-lead electrocardiogram

recommendations which simply refer to the need to carry out such evaluation on the first and second visits.

The recommendations for laboratory investigations in uncomplicated hypertension are remarkably concordant (*Table 2.1*). The only dissentient recommendation is the explicit exclusion of urinary microscopy in the British guidelines, presumably on the grounds of low yield of relevant information. It should be noted that the evidence for the advice on laboratory investigations is rated D in the Canadian report, i.e. it is based upon expert opinion rather than clinical trials. The basis for the recommendations is clearly an assessment of net benefit when possible impact upon management is set against cost. There is remarkably little epidemiological or trial data to provide guidance. Under the circumstances, expert groups have understandably elected for the view that only the cheapest and least invasive investigations should be recommended routinely. In the case of forms of secondary hypertension, such as primary aldosteronism, as has been pointed out above, this is critically dependent upon controversial data on prevalence. In the case of echocardiography to assess left ventricular mass, a cost–benefit analysis assessing the likelihood of impact upon management would seem to be critically important but it is not used to support recommendations. This is not a defect confined to expert committees. The volume of research devoted to designing and testing pharmacological treatment is not matched by the number of studies on other aspects of patient management.[20]

Assessment of blood pressure

All the guidelines emphasize the importance of correct clinical procedures for measurement under standardized conditions with reasonable agreement over what these are. Two additional techniques are now available: ambulatory and home monitoring.

Defining the indications for ambulatory blood pressure monitoring (ABPM) presents a significant challenge in the absence of relevant trial data. The stronger association between ABPM and target-organ damage as compared with that between clinic blood pressures and target-organ damage is well established. It is probable, although not proven, that ABPM provides superior prognostic data for cardiovascular morbidity and mortality. Unfortunately, there is no end-point trial evidence to guide treatment decisions comparable to that available for clinic blood pressures, and ABPM values are usually significantly lower than these. As a result, there is uncertainty about both the level of ambulatory blood pressure at which drug treatment should be recommended and the blood pressure levels that represent optimal control. Pooled values for ABPM in healthy individuals have yielded a 95th percentile value of 138/87 mmHg.[21] On the basis of such studies, JNC VI takes a daytime mean of <135/85 mmHg as 'normal'. On the other hand, the WHO–ISH guidelines define a normal clinic blood pressure as <130/85 mmHg and an optimal blood pressure as <120/80 mmHg. Since the average difference between ABPM and clinic blood pressure is 12/7 mmHg, this definition would result in far more blood pressures defined as abnormal on ABPM.

Such references to 'normality' and 'abnormality', so out of line with Pickering's definition of hypertension as a 'quantitative deviation from the mean',[22] reflect the absence of information about risk for any given ambulatory pressure. Normality provides the only feasible alternative way of classifying data but it is clinically unhelpful. In particular, it makes it difficult to reconcile ABPM measurements with the strategy of quantitative cardiovascular risk assessment. As a result, none of the guidelines recommends routine use of ABPM. All suggest unusual blood pressure variability, apparent resistance to drug treatment, symptoms suggestive of hypotension and suspicion of 'white-coat hypertension' as indications. The latter provides a clinical conundrum which none of the guidelines completely resolves. How does one distinguish such patients in whom clinic blood pressures are elevated? The traditional solution is to identify those with no evidence of target-organ damage. Unfortunately, clinical evidence of this is rare in patients with milder degrees of hypertension, particularly if echocardiographic screening for left ventricular hypertrophy is not carried out. The British guidelines provide a pragmatic approach by considering as eligible only those patients in whom ABPM may alter management. This clearly excludes those whose overall cardiovascular risk places them below the threshold for drug treatment, or those whose overall risk from target-organ damage or complications puts them in the treatment category independently of blood pressure. On the other hand, there is a group of patients with higher blood pressure levels

(>160/100 mmHg) who have few other risk factors and whose overall cardiovascular risk would otherwise place them below the treatment level. Normal blood pressures by ABPM would alter that decision. Such patients are likely to be only a small proportion of the hypertensive population according to the calculations of Haq et al.[23]

Data on the clinical and prognostic value of home blood pressure monitoring is much weaker than for ABPM and none of the guidelines recommends it for routine use. On the other hand, it has the advantage of being cheaper and involving the patient more in their own management. On these grounds, the WHO–ISH and Canadian recommendations, and JNC VI tentatively, suggest that it may be useful in patients suspected of being non-compliant, as well as for patients in whom ABPM may be otherwise indicated.

Period of observation

All guidelines suggest monitoring of blood pressure before starting drug therapy in patients who are not at high cardiovascular risk. This serves several purposes:

(a) to allow blood pressure to fall to usual values as a result of habituation and regression to the mean;
(b) to obtain more blood pressure readings to improve risk assessment;
(c) to assess the efficacy of lifestyle modifications.

Although the length of the observation period differs (*Table 2.2*), the discrepancies are more apparent than real, since all the recommendations relate the duration of observation to the risk level, although some (JNC VI and WHO–ISH) are much more prescriptive about this relationship than the others.

The observation period is curtailed in patients at higher risk and early treatment recommended. The degree of curtailment varies and the recommendations exhibit some curious paradoxes. Thus, JNC VI recommends early drug therapy (after 1 week to 1 month of observation) in

Table 2.2   Duration of observation period in lower risk patients before pharmacological treatment is started

	Observation period (months)
British	4–6
Canadian	6
JNC VI	1–12
New Zealand	6
WHO–ISH	3–12

patients with blood pressures >160/100 mmHg. The WHO–ISH guidelines recommend values of >180/110 mmHg in the absence of other risk factors. The Canadian recommendations imply a value >180/105 mmHg, while the British guidelines are the most conservative in recommending a value of >200/110 mmHg; the New Zealand guidelines give no specific advice about curtailing the observation period.

The anomaly in these recommendations is that higher blood pressures, in isolation, without additional risk factors (especially age) may carry quite a low absolute risk. Most non-smoking men and women with a blood pressure of 160/100 mmHg, between the ages of 30 and 50, will have an absolute risk of a cardiovascular event of <2% (which is the threshold absolute risk for drug treatment in the British guidelines for patients with lower blood pressure levels). Application of these guidelines would, therefore, result in some patients with high initial pressures receiving early drug treatment who would not merit drug treatment at all on the basis of overall cardiovascular risk.

Lifestyle modifications

The Canadian guidelines for lifestyle modification are unique in that they are based upon a separate series of reports derived from systematic reviews of the literature.[24] As such, they provide a valuable assessment of the magnitude of the blood pressure-lowering effect that can be expected. All guidelines recommend weight reduction, moderation of alcohol intake in heavy drinkers, regular physical activity and moderation of dietary sodium, together with increased fruit and vegetable intake, and reduced total and saturated fat intake. The latter is mainly aimed at dyslipidaemia, although the recently completed Dietary Approach to Stopping Hypertension (DASH) study suggested a valuable blood pressure-lowering action additional to that produced by fruit and vegetables.[25] The WHO–ISH guidelines additionally recommend an increased intake of fish. There is less agreement about psychological interventions such as relaxation and biofeedback. Most guidelines are sceptical about claims for a specific effect on blood pressure. Only the Canadian guidelines recommend cognitive behaviour modification in individual patients 'to reduce the negative effects of stress'.

Threshold risk for drug therapy

Previous guidelines differed on the level of risk at which pharmacological treatment was recommended, the selection of first-line drugs and on the level of blood pressure which should be targeted. There are still significant differences on the first two issues, while opinion has converged substantially on the last. Social values play a major role in the first of these, while the residual differences about the second and third largely reflect scientific uncertainties.

Guidelines have all moved towards an approach that requires assessment of total cardiovascular risk. None has yet taken the final step of applying this approach to all strata of blood pressure, as has been pointed out, in relation to the duration of the observation period. Two sets of guidelines adopt a fully quantitative approach using epidemiological calculation of risk – the New Zealand and the British guidelines – both confining it to mild to moderate hypertension. Above a specified level of sustained pressure (170/100 mmHg in the former and 159/99 mmHg in the latter) pharmacological treatment is recommended independently of risk profile. This results in the same anomalies as those seen in relation to the duration of observation period. Many patients who have a calculated 10-year risk of a cardiovascular event, well below the 20% level which is used for mild hypertension, will be treated because their blood pressure exceeds these arbitrary thresholds. The use of blood pressure as an overriding criterion for drug treatment in these patients would seem to reflect a reluctance to abandon completely the approach adopted by earlier guidelines, which used other risk factors only to lower the threshold pressure at which treatment was indicated. The Canadian recommendations are closest to this historical position as a result of their reliance upon intervention trials rather than epidemiological data. Drug therapy is recommended for all blood pressures ≥160/100 mmHg and for pressures below this level in the presence of other risk factors. JNC VI and the WHO guidelines both adopt a semi-quantitative approach. Patients are categorized in different risk categories according to blood pressure level and the number and nature of other risk factors (*Table 2.3*).

The WHO–ISH guidelines recommend drug treatment with varying degrees of urgency for all patients in the medium- to very high-risk categories and to patients with sustained blood pressures of 150/95 mmHg or more in the low-risk category. JNC VI uses a matrix based upon three blood pressure strata (high–normal, Stage 1 and Stage 2) and three risk groups (for risk factors other than blood pressure, target-organ damage or established cardiovascular disease). It recommends drug treatment for all patients with blood pressures ≥140/90 mmHg, although only after an observation period of 1 year in the lowest risk categories.

The risk threshold selected plays a critical role on the proportion of the population who will receive pharmacological treatment on the basis of their recommendations, although this question assumes especial importance in the elderly. None of the guidelines presents this information for different age strata. Because lower levels of blood pressure approach the mode of the blood pressure distribution curve and progressively lower levels of cardiovascular risk recruit more eligible candidates for treatment exponentially, numerically quite small differences in risk or

Table 2.3 Categorization of risk in the WHO–ISH guidelines

	Blood pressure (mmHg)		
	Grade 1 (mild hypertension) SBP 140–159 mmHg or DBP 90–99 mmHg	Grade 2 (moderate hypertension) SBP 160–179 mmHg or DBP 100–109 mmHg	Grade 3 (severe hypertension) SBP >180 mmHg or DBP >110 mmHg
No other risk factors	Low risk	Medium risk	High risk
One to two risk factors	Medium risk	Medium risk	Very high risk
Three or more risk factors or target-organ damage or diabetes	High risk	High risk	Very high risk
Accelerated clinical conditions†	Very high risk	Very high risk	Very high risk

*SBP, systolic blood pressure; DBP, diastolic blood pressure. †For example, established cerebrovascular, ischaemic heart disease, cardiac failure, renal failure or accelerated hypertension.

blood pressure threshold can have a major impact on the numbers recommended for treatment. In 1996, Fahey and Peters[26] applied the then current guidelines to a population of British hypertensive patients in primary care. The percentage of patients with treated, controlled blood pressure, according to the various guidelines, ranged from 17.5 (JNC V) to 84.6% (Canadian). Although there has been some convergence in recommendations since then, the application of current guidelines would continue to show major divergences.

Use of absolute risk

JNC VI makes no statement about the absolute risk level the guidelines target, although it directs readers to appropriate epidemiological databases. The WHO–ISH report provides a rather wide range of absolute 10-year risk of cardiovascular events for each of its risk categories. It is easy to obtain more precise values by applying the New Zealand risk chart to the different categories of hypertension in JNC VI and WHO–ISH. Adhering to their advice will result in some patients at quite low 10-year risk receiving medication. This will happen more often with the JNC VI recommendations than in the case of WHO–ISH. In younger uncomplicated hypertensives, the estimate may be less than five cardiovascular events per 100 patients over 10 years. By employing higher blood pressure thresholds for treatment independent of the presence of other risk factors, the British and New Zealand guidelines will result in fewer very low-risk patients receiving treatment, but at the expense of more explicit inconsistency between patients who are subject to full, rigorous risk profiling and those who are not.

The difficulties which inevitably emerge as a result of the movement to absolute individual risk as a major criterion of treatment raise a number of major issues. The debate over these is likely to grow over the next few years.

Use of risk tables in practice

The first concern is logistic and probably the simplest to resolve. Doctors are demonstrably poor at assessing cardiovascular risk in hypertensives, which they consistently overestimate in younger patients. Even the semi-quantitative charts employed in JNC VI and the WHO–ISH guidelines are unlikely to be memorized, particularly by non-hypertension specialists who have many other conditions to evaluate. The New Zealand and British charts manifestly require access to printed information or software. For most professionals, the need to consult such sources of information may require a significant change in their normal practice. This is not in itself an undesirable consequence of guideline evolution. The limited amount of research evidence on methods for improving the implementation of guidelines for treating hypertension suggests that patient-specific reminders at the time of consultation may result in improvement.[27]

Transferability of absolute risk calculations

The British and New Zealand tables use the Framingham data for risk calculation. While this is probably acceptable for relative risk assessment, it is clear that the Framingham function overestimates coronary heart disease risk in some other populations, e.g. the French, Hawaiians and Israelis.[28] Haq *et al.*[28] compared the Framingham assessment with the Munster (PROCAM), Dundee and British Regional Heart risk functions when applied to a British hypertensive population. There was good agreement for average risk but considerable disparities in the evaluation of individual risk when the Dundee and British Regional Heart functions were applied. There was, however, an acceptable degree of agreement between the Framingham and PROCAM risk assessment. These data were the only two which included measurement of high-density lipoprotein cholesterol, suggesting that the sophistication of risk profiling rather than epidemiological differences in the cohort populations studied were responsible. Thus, it seems likely that the application of Framingham data to British, German and probably northern European populations, as well as North Americans, is valid. This cannot be assumed for other populations, especially those with a lower incidence of coronary heart disease, such as subjects from the Mediterranean littoral.

Role of judgemental values

Absolute risks are theoretically calculable 'hard' scientific data. However, the ultimate objective of treatment is not to target risk but to achieve benefit. Individual benefit from blood pressure reduction is not, however, identical with reversal of risk, although it is often treated as though it were simply the reciprocal. Thus, for instance the 'number needed to treat' is often used to compare the value of different interventions. In isolation, this statistic is an insufficient basis on which to make a decision. Benefit implies a value judgement. How important to the individual or to society is the prevention of disability or death? How are the needs of the two balanced? This becomes a critical judgement when resources are a limiting factor in the availability of treatment. Such concerns explain the strong reaction which the New Zealand guidelines provoked when they pioneered the use of risk factor tables. Begg *et al.*[29] refer to 'unacceptable anomalies' in the use of a 5-year absolute risk as a guide to treatment. 'It equates 5 years of life in a 70-year-old with 5 years in a 30-year-old. It also equates the impact of a stroke in a 70-year-old with a stroke in a 30-year-old'. Echoing identical concerns, Simpson[30] suggested that a

factor should be built in to risk calculation to allow for the greater importance of morbidity or mortality in a younger patient with many years of
active life ahead. No doubt such considerations were influential in the
decision to set an absolute threshold level for blood pressure above
which treatment was recommended, independent of risk. This, however,
is clearly only a partial solution to the problem. Another suggestion is to
use actuarial life expectancy rather than 5- or 10-year risk of cardiovascular events as a basis for treatment.[31] So far, no guidelines committees
have take up the challenge.

Costs of treating and not treating

Much of the discussion about the use of absolute risk confuses two separate issues about the balance of treatment in the young and the elderly:
value of health and life to the individual and the economic cost to society
of treating a large proportion of the population. Since both systolic blood
pressure and cardiovascular risk rise progressively with age, the use of
single threshold values for either will result in the inclusion of progressively more patients in the treatment category. Indeed, with the exception
of the Canadian guidelines, which retain a high threshold blood pressure
value in the elderly (160/105 mmHg), all the guidelines reviewed here
would result in treatment of the majority of the elderly population (>65
years of age) if adhered to rigorously. These concerns led the previously
mentioned reference to two levels of risk in the British guidelines. The
lower level (20% 10-year cardiovascular risk) was recommended 'as
resources allow'. Other guidelines, which also eschew detailed economic
analysis, do not confront this issue directly. There is a fallacy in the
resource argument as applied to the elderly. The total cost to society of
managing the consequences of hypertension in the elderly population
greatly exceeds the costs of blood pressure control.[18] A formal analysis
of cost-effectiveness taking account of strokes and myocardial infarcts
attributable to hypertension concluded that treatment of mild hypertension in the elderly resulted in minimal net cost or an actual financial
return.[32] This leads to the inevitable conclusion that the debate about the
consequences of recommendations based rigidly upon absolute risk
should focus on the important, and occasionally emotive, question of
whether such guidelines are too restrictive in their recommendations for
younger patients.

Role of early or late intervention in preventing complications

While social values and economic cost play a major role in these discus-
sions, the answer to this latter question lies in traditional epidemiology
and pathophysiology. End-point data derived from trials of a few years
duration and 5- or 10-year epidemiological risk of an event may seriously

underestimate the longer term consequences of quite modest blood pressure elevation two or three decades later. On these grounds (among others), JNC VI, for instance, stated that the committee had 'extrapolated treatment effects beyond duration of the clinical trials, based on physiological and epidemiological data'. The insurance data from pretreatment days provide some relevant evidence. The life expectancy of a man aged 35 (41 years) was 8.5 years shorter compared with the population average when his blood pressure was 140/95 mmHg and shorter by 16 years (39%) when his blood pressure was 140/100 mmHg. In the absence of other risk factors, even the latter blood pressure level would place his 10-year risk of a cardiovascular event at <1%. The New Zealand guidelines would not suggest drug treatment for such an individual although the British guidelines would, on the basis of a diastolic pressure of 100 mmHg, although not if it had been 99 mmHg. Would later intervention, when such a patient entered the recommended drug treatment category, reverse these risks to the same extent as it would if treatment had been given earlier? This seems unlikely in the case of ischaemic heart disease where trial data shows a shortfall in reversal of epidemiological risk, although there are other explanations of this phenomenon.[33]

Cardiac failure attributable to hypertension provides other evidence. The most frequently cited meta-analysis of intervention trials[33] does not include cardiac failure as a separate end-point, neither did it figure in the earlier trials in younger subjects (excluding the Veterans trial).[34] Cardiac failure is, however, overwhelmingly a disease of the elderly and meta-analysis of trials in these patients shows a reduction greater than that calculated for coronary heart disease and stoke.[35] However, it is clear from the Framingham data that cardiac structural and functional changes that were associated with the later development of cardiac failure occurred decades before.[36] The benefits of treatment in preventing such consequences are not deducible from trial data in younger subjects.

None of this evidence is conclusive and it seems improbable that randomized controlled trials of sufficiently prolonged duration will ever be carried out. The danger is that guidelines drawn up on the basis of a very narrow view of evidence-based medicine, which give absolute priority to such trials over other sources of evidence, will draw misleading conclusions which ignore their limitations.[37] Encouragement by governments and health-care funders to adopt this form of evidence-based approach on the grounds that it will save cost can only make matters worse.

Drug selection

There are clinical indications and contraindications to individual classes of drugs in specific clinical situations. Thus, angiotensin-converting-enzyme (ACE) inhibitors should be used in patients with cardiac failure or type 1 diabetes and proteinuria, but not in pregnant patients. Alpha blockers have useful additional benefits in patients with prostatism. Likewise, diuretics are to be best avoided in patients with gout and β-blockers certainly in asthmatics. Although guidelines differ in the degree of emphasis they place upon indications and contra-indications, there are not, unsurprisingly major differences of opinion. However, guidelines continue to diverge on the choice of initial treatment when such factors do not apply. There are three relevant issues, only two of which are addressed in published guidelines.

Actions additional to blood pressure lowering

The major point of contention centres on the importance attached to end-point trial data demonstrating efficacy. Those who demand such evidence are opposed by those who argue that it is safe to assume that blood pressure lowering *per se* is responsible for the beneficial effect of treatment upon cardiovascular events. The former would confine the choice to diuretics, β-blockers and, most recently, ACE inhibitors; although, in the case of the latter, the relevant trial data were published too late to influence any of the guidelines with the exception of the Canadian recommendations. The possibility that some newer classes of agent have particularly beneficial haemodynamic actions or specific pharmacological effects inhibiting, for instance, atherogenesis has been endlessly debated on the basis of experimental observations. There is, however, a lack of trial evidence, although large intervention trials currently being carried out will undoubtedly throw light on this question.

Economic considerations

The second consideration is the role of cost in drug selection. Predictably, the British guidelines are most forthright in stating that 'the least expensive drug, with the most supportive trial evidence [a low dose of thiazide diuretic] should be preferred'. The New Zealand guidelines make the same recommendation with explicit reference to the cost of bendrofluazide, although they do not define what role this played in their decision. Both JNC VI (which elects for thiazide diuretics or β-blockers) and the WHO–ISH guidelines (which regards all classes of drug as suitable) refer to the importance of economic factors in the final decision. The Canadian guidelines, consistent with their policy of ignoring economic cost and giving priority to end-point trial data, recommend a diuretic, β-blocker or ACE inhibitor. The question of cost cannot, of course, be dissociated from the debate on risk reversal. A greater impact on, say, coronary heart disease would have a major effect upon cost–benefit analysis.

Effect of changes in medication on persistence with treatment

There is another assumption in guideline recommendations that is not made explicitly but which is important in drug selection. It has to be assumed that intolerance or inadequate control over the initial period of treatment has no subsequent deleterious effects. This seems justifiable in the case of later cardiovascular events, but there is evidence that treatment failure or intolerance does have an influence on a patient's persistence with treatment. Thus, a prescription monitoring study carried out in Saskatchewan reported that a single drug change in a 6-month period of treatment was associated with a 7% fall in persistence with treatment, while two or more changes were associated with a 25% fall.[38] This is indirect evidence in a field where research is scanty. It does, however, serve to underline the argument that drug tolerance and efficacy in blood pressure lowering may play a role in drug selection quite independently of trial evidence for long-term effects upon cardiovascular events.

Target blood pressure

Only one trial has specifically addressed the issue of the optimal blood pressure that should be targeted – the Hypertension Optimal Treatment (HOT) trial.[39] This showed no difference in outcome between the three randomized diastolic pressure target groups (<90, 85 or 80 mmHg), although target groups showed only modest differences of 2 mmHg in achieved blood pressure. Strictly, therefore, HOT only suggests the absence of harm as a result of targeting diastolic blood pressure to the lower strata. A retrospective on treatment analysis demonstrated minimal events with a blood pressure of 139/83 mmHg. In spite of residual uncertainties, there has nevertheless been a gratifying, if partial, convergence of advice in the most recent versions of established guidelines, no doubt influenced by the powerful epidemiological evidence for continuity of risk (*Table 2.4*). In the light of stronger trial evidence, most guidelines now emphasize the importance of particular tight blood pressure control in one specific high-risk group – the diabetic hypertensive (*Table 2.4*)

The systolic target for blood pressure is a particularly ambitious one, as is shown by the failure to achieve systolic targets in a number of studies of blood pressure control in clinical practice. While professional conservatism in emphasizing diastolic rather than systolic pressure may play a role in this, the failure to achieve systolic control in many patients, both in specialist clinics and in clinical trials, suggests a genuine resistance. Both JNC VI and the WHO–ISH guidelines classify such patients as suffering from 'refractory hypertension' and go on to list causes amongst which non-adherence to therapy figures prominently. This is difficult to establish with certainty, but it is often misleading and sometimes danger-

Table 2.4   Target blood pressures recommended for treated hypertension

Guideline	Essential hypertension		Diabetic hypertension	
	SBP* (mmHg)	DBP† (mmHg)	SBP* (mmHg)	DBP† (mmHg)
British	<140	<85	<140	<80
Canadian	<140	<90	<130	<80
JNC VI	<140 or lower if tolerated	<90 or lower if tolerated	<130	<85
New Zealand	–	<90	–	–
WHO–ISH	<130	<85	<130	<85
Older patients	<140	<90		

*SBP, systolic blood pressure; †DBP, diastolic blood pressure.

ous to attribute failure to achieve systolic goals to such specific causes. False expectations of what can be achieved, particularly in the older patient with systolic hypertension, can have harmful consequences for patient care. The British guidelines are more open about this when they state that: 'Despite best practice, these levels will be difficult to achieve in some hypertensive people'.

Conclusions

The gestation of guidelines for hypertension has frequently been a painful one. Accusations of hidden agendas, misrepresentation and naivety have been accompanied by stories of walkouts and resignations from expert committees. This is to be expected when, in the face of partial evidence, scientific conclusions are intermingled with often implicit judgements of cost and value. Although there are logical inconsistencies in recommendations, it is worth emphasizing that there is now a fair consensus on the overall plan of treatment. The question of who should be treated has tended to assume greater importance in setting recent guidelines apart from each other rather than the equally important question of how they should be treated. The danger in addressing all these issues is to forget the main objective, i.e. to set a framework of good practice within which there is room for genuine differences of opinion and the individual preferences of the patient and the doctor. Succumbing to the temptation to produce ever more detailed and prescriptive recommendations while paying lip service to the latter is no solution.

References

1. World Health Organization–International Society of Hypertension (WHO–ISH) Guidelines for the Management of Hypertension. J Hypertens 1999; 17: 151–183.

2. Ramsay LE, Williams B, Johnston GD et al. Guidelines for management of hypertension: report of the third working party of the British Hypertension Society. J Hum Hypertens 1999; 13: 569–592.

3. Feldman RD, Campbell N, Larochelle P et al. Canadian recommendations for the management of hypertension. CMAJ 1999; 161 (suppl 12) S1–S39.

4. Joint National Committee on Prevention, Detection, Evaluation and Treatment of High Blood Pressure. The sixth report. Arch Intern Med 1997; 157: 2413–2445.

5. Mabadeje AF. WHO–ISH guidelines for the management of hypertension: implementation in Africa – the Nigerian experience. Clin Exp Hypertens 1999; 21: 671–681.

6. Opie LH, Steyn K. Rationale for the hypertension guidelines for primary care in South Africa. S Afr Med J 1995; 85: 1325–1328, 1330–1331.

7. Unwin N, Mugusi F, Aspray T et al. Tackling the emerging endemic of non-communicable diseases in sub-Saharan Africa: the essential NCD health intervention project. Public Health 1999; 113: 141–146.

8. Kassirer JP. The quality of care and the quality of measuring it. N Engl J Med 1993; 339: 1263–1265.

9. Swales JD. Critical assessment of hypertension guidelines. In: Oparil S, Weber MA, eds. Hypertension: a companion to Brenner and Rector's the kidney. WB Saunders Company: Philadelphia, PA, 1999, 375–382.

10. Core Services Committee. The management of mildly raised blood pressure in New Zealand 1995. Core Services Committee PO Box 5013, Wellington, New Zealand.

11. Anon. The management of hypertension: a consensus statement. Med J Aust 1994; 160 (suppl): S1–S16.

12. Feder G. Clinical guidelines in 1994. Lets be careful out there. BMJ 1994; 309: 1457–1458.

13. Ramsay LE, Williams B, Johnston GD et al. British Hypertension Society guidelines for hypertension management: Summary. BMJ 1999; 319: 630–635.

14. Carruthers SG, Larochelle P, Haynes RB et al. Report of the Canadian Hypertension Society Consensus Conference: 1. Introduction. CMAJ 1993; 149: 289–293.

15. EBM Working Group. Evidence-based medicine. JAMA 1992; 268: 2420–2425.

16. Swales JD. Evidence-based medicine and hypertension. J Hypertens 1999; 17: 1511–1516.

17. Gordon RD, Stowasser M, Klemm SA, Tunny TJ. Primary aldosteronism and other forms of mineralocorticoid hypertension. In: Swales JD, ed. Textbook of hypertension. Blackwell Scientific Publications: Oxford, UK, 1994, 865–892.

18. Swales JD. The costs of not treating hypertension. Blood Press 1999; 8: 1–2.

19. Expert Committee on the Diagnosis and Classification of Diabetes. Diabetes Care 1997; 20: 1183–1197.

20. Swales JD. Research and devel-

opment in the NHS. J Roy Soc Med 1998; 91 (suppl 36): 18–20.

21. O'Brien E, Staessen JA. What is 'hypertension'? Lancet 1999; 353: 1541–1542.

22. Swales JD, ed. Platt versus Pickering: an episode in recent medical history. London: The Keynes Press, 1985.

23. Haq IU, Wallis EJ, Yeo WW et al. The impact of ambulatory blood pressure on estimation of cardiovascular risk. J Hypertens 1997; 15: 1540–1541.

24. Campbell NRC, Burgews, E, Choi BCK et al. Lifestyle modifications to prevent and control hypertension: methods and overview of the Canadian recommendations. CMAJ 1999; 160 (suppl 9): S1–S6.

25. Appel LJ, Moore TJ, Obarzanek E et al. A clinical trial of the effects of dietary patterns on blood pressure. N Engl J Med 1997; 336: 1117–1124.

26. Fahey TP, Peters TJ. What constitutes controlled hypertension? Patient-based comparison of hypertension guidelines. BMJ 1996; 313: 93–96.

27. Ebrahim S. Detection, adherence and control of hypertension for the prevention of stroke: a systematic review. Health Technology Assessment 1998; 2.

28. Haq IU, Ramsay LE, Yeo WW et al. Is the Framingham risk function valid for northern European populations? A comparison of methods for estimating absolute coronary risk in high risk men. Heart 1999; 81: 40–46.

29. Begg EJ, Nicholls MG, Richards AM. The management of mildly raised blood pressure in New Zealand: an alternative view. N Z Med J 1996; 109: 237–240.

30. Simpson FO. Guidelines for antihypertensive therapy: problems with a strategy based on absolute risk. J Hypertens 1996; 14: 683–689.

31. Swales JD. Treating hypertension. J Hypertens 1996; 14: 813–815.

32. Johannesson M. The cost-effectiveness of hypertension treatment in Sweden. Pharmacoeconomics 1995; 7: 242–250.

33. Collins R, Peto R. Antihypertensive drug therapy: effects on stroke and coronary heart disease. In: Swales JD, ed. Textbook of hypertension. Blackwell Scientific Publications: Oxford, UK, 1994, 1156–1164.

34. Veterans Administration Cooperative Study Group on Antihypertensive Agents. Effects of treatment on morbidity in hypertension. JAMA 1967; 202: 116–122.

35. Cutler JA, Psarty BM, MacMahon S, Furberg CD. Public health issues in hypertensive control: what has been learned from clinical trials? In: Laragh JH, Brenner BM, eds. Hypertension: pathophysiology, diagnosis and management. Raven Press: New York, 1995, 253–272.

36. Levy D, Larson MG, Vasan R et al. The progression from hypertension to congestive heart failure. JAMA 1996; 275: 1557–1562.

37. Swales JD. Evidence-based medicine and hypertension. J Hypertens 1999; 17: 1511–1516.

38. Caro JJ, Speckman JL, Salas M. The effect of initial drug choice on persistence with antihypertensive therapy: the importance of actual practice data. CMAJ 1999; 160: 41–46.

39. Hansson L, Zanchetti A, Carruthers SG et al. Effect of intensive blood pressure lowering and low dose aspirin in patients with hypertension: principle results of the Hypertension Optimal Treatment (HOT) randomised trial. Lancet 1998; 351: 1755–1762.

3
Treatment of diabetic hypertension: goals and choices

Peter D Hart and George L Bakris

Introduction

Hypertension is prevalent in individuals with diabetes, particularly when nephropathy is present. It is approximately twice as common in people with type 2 diabetes as in those without,[1,2] and coexists with diabetes in up to 85% of those with type 2 diabetes who have diabetic nephropathy.[3] Diabetes is the most common cause of end-stage renal disease in the USA and over 90% have coexistent hypertension.[4]

Hypertension exacerbates all of the vascular complications of diabetes including renal disease, coronary heart disease, stroke, peripheral vascular disease, lower extremity amputations and retinopathy. Moreover, people with both diabetes and hypertension have a five- to sixfold greater risk of developing end-stage renal disease compared to people with hypertension and no evidence of diabetes.[1] Patients with both diabetes and hypertension not only have a higher incidence of renal disease but also a greater prevalence of cardiovascular risk factors including dyslipidemia, microalbuminuria, hyperuricemia, a thrombotic tendency and left ventricular hypertrophy.[1] It should be appreciated that the most common cause of death in people with diabetic nephropathy is secondary to cardiovascular causes. Moreover, the risk of a cardiovascular event in patients with diabetes and no prior history of myocardial infarction is similar to that of people without diabetes who have had a previous myocardial infarction.[5]

The incidence of end-stage renal disease due to diabetes continues to rise, despite increased awareness and recommendations for preventive strategies developed by various public health organizations. Over the past two decades there has been a relentless increase in those starting dialysis in the USA, primarily related to diabetes (*Fig. 3.1*). Factors implicated in this increased incidence include the continual rise in new cases of diabetes, poor patient education and adherence to prescribed medications, and failure to achieve goal blood pressure.

Several studies in patients with renal insufficiency clearly document

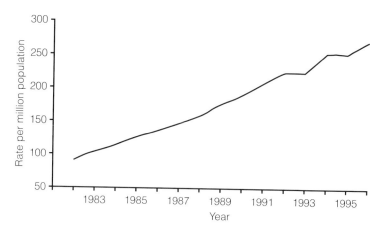

Figure 3.1

Incidence of reported renal replacement therapy, 1982–1997, based on USRDS 1999 annual report, adjusted for age, race and sex. Reprinted with permission from Bakris *et al.*[15]

that lower levels of blood pressure result in slower rates of decline in renal function.[6-8] This observation was confirmed in a retrospective analysis of clinical trials in people with renal insufficiency resulting from diabetes as well as other etiologies.[9] In this analysis, it was clear that an achieved systolic blood pressure that was 10 mmHg lower (134 versus 144 mmHg) translated into an additional slowing of renal disease progression by an average of 4 ml per minute per year – decline rates of 7 versus 3 ml per minute per year. Thus, someone of 50 years of age with a glomerular filtration rate of 50 ml per minute and a systolic blood pressure averaging 144 mmHg would be on dialysis about 8 years earlier than someone with a systolic blood pressure of 134 mmHg.

Proteinuria is the hallmark of renal disease in diabetes and is now recognized as an independent risk factor for cardiovascular disease.[10] The stage before proteinuria i.e. microalbuminuria, is associated much more with an increased cardiovascular risk and predicts nephropathy progression in type 1 diabetes. Indeed, a recent study demonstrated a strong, linear relationship between the severity of angiographic coronary artery disease and the degree of albuminuria.[11] This relationship was present in all patients but was most pronounced in those with diabetes. The National Kidney Foundation PARADE task force has reviewed the evidence relating proteinuria and microalbuminuria to renal and cardiovascular risk. Screening for microalbuminuria is recommended in patients with diabetes but also for others at increased risk for renal or cardiovascular diseases. If proteinuria or microalbuminuria is present then further diagnostic testing may be warranted, and aggressive risk-factor modification is recommended.[10]

Until recently, reductions in proteinuria had not been clearly associated with renal benefit. Now, however, there are numerous long-term clinical trials available in patients who have lost >35% of their renal function, with or without diabetes, demonstrating that reductions in proteinuria of >30% below baseline correlate with marked reductions in renal disease progression.[12] The PARADE initiative included an analysis of different levels of proteinuria and their impact on renal disease progression. This, in turn, led to the PARADE recommendation that therapies used to treat blood pressure should also target reductions in proteinuria.[10]

Blood pressure goal

Diagnosis

Accurate measurements of blood pressure is mandatory to establish the diagnosis of hypertension. The key steps that should be followed include: (a) patients should be seated in a chair with their back supported, and their arms bared and supported at heart level; (b) measurement should begin after 5 minutes of rest, palpation of the radial pulse and use of an appropriate cuff size; (c) two or more blood pressure readings, separated by 2 minutes, should be taken and averaged.

Goal

The sixth report of the Joint National Committee on Detection, Evaluation, and Treatment of High Blood Pressure (JNC VI) recommends the initiation of antihypertensive drug therapy in all diabetic patients with a blood pressure >130/85 mmHg.[13] This strategy goes beyond treating established hypertension (i.e. blood pressure ≥140/90 mmHg) to treating high normal blood pressure (defined as 130–139/85–89 mmHg) in diabetic patients.

There is overwhelming evidence from epidemiological data that supports the need for a lower blood pressure and a more intensive blood pressure control in diabetics with hypertension. Over the past 5 years, additional long-term clinical trials not only support these recommendations but also form the basis to support an even lower level of blood pressure than that proposed by the JNC VI guidelines. A blood pressure level of 130/80 mmHg in patients with diabetes is supported by these recent trials. This blood pressure goal was adopted by the Canadian Hypertension Society in 1999.[14] More recently, the National Kidney Foundation and the American Diabetes Association have also adopted the <130/80 mmHg blood pressure goal.[15,16] An analysis of long-term clinical trials, e.g. the Modification of Diet in Renal Disease (MDRD) trial that evaluated the rate of decline in renal function at a randomized level of blood pressure, demonstrate that the lower the blood pressure then the greater the preservation of renal function.[6,17] Moreover, in a retrospective analysis of the MDRD trial, those who had >1 g per day of proteinuria and renal insufficiency, regardless of etiology, had slower rates of renal disease progression when the blood pressure was <125/75 mmHg.[18]

The first trial to show the benefit of a lower than usual blood pressure goal in reducing cardiovascular events in the subgroup of people with diabetes was the Hypertension Optimal Treatment (HOT) trial.[19] In this study, 1501 diabetic patients were randomized to one of three diastolic blood pressure targets: <90, <85, or <80 mmHg. Initial antihypertensive therapy in this group was with the calcium-channel blocker (CCB) felodipine. However, 73% of the people randomized to the lowest blood pressure group required approximately 2.7 different antihypertensive medications and 40% of the patients in this group also received an angiotensin-converting-enzyme (ACE) inhibitor. An important finding in this study was that those who achieved the lowest diastolic blood pressure (<80 mmHg) also experienced the lowest rate of cardiovascular events. Additionally, a much higher percentage of those with an average blood pressure of <130/85 mmHg had no elevations in serum creatinine at follow-up compared to those with higher pressures.

Another study that showed the long-term benefit of a lower than usual blood pressure goal for people with diabetes was the United Kingdom Prospective Diabetes Study (UKPDS) 38.[20] In this study, 1148 type 2 diabetics were randomized to one of two goal blood pressures: <150/85 mmHg (the 'intensively treated' group) or <180/105 mmHg (the 'conventional' group), and followed for an average of 8.4 years. When the study was completed, those randomized to the intensively treated group benefited from 32% fewer deaths, 44% fewer strokes, 24% fewer diabetes-related end-points (including amputations) and 37% fewer microvascular complications (including retinal hemorrhages). The intensively treated group had an average blood pressure of 144/82 mmHg, while the control group was only slightly higher at 154/87 mmHg – a difference of only 5 mmHg in diastolic blood pressure and 10 mmHg in systolic blood pressure. Thus, tight blood pressure control (defined as a blood pressure <150/85 mmHg) resulted in a significant risk reduction of diabetes-related morbidity and mortality compared to less intensive blood pressure control.

Similarly, in the HOT trial there was also a 4 mmHg difference in the achieved diastolic blood pressure between the intensively treated group and other target groups (84.6 versus 81 mmHg). Even these small reductions in blood pressure resulted in a significantly lower cardiovascular event rate in the diabetes subgroup and a greater preservation of renal function in the intensively treated group. Thus, data from the HOT and UKPDS 38 trials indicate that a reduction in diastolic blood pressure by as little as 5 mmHg results in a significant reduction in diabetes-related cardiovascular and renal injury. Additionally, in the UKPDS 38 trial, a comparison of tight blood pressure control versus tight glucose control revealed that, in type 2 diabetics, blood pressure control led to a relatively greater cardiovascular risk reduction than did tight blood glucose control (*Fig. 3.2*). Thus, reducing blood pressure to the suggested lower goal of 130/80 mmHg is critical for preserving not only renal function but also for reducing cardiovascular injury.

In summary, these trials, as well as the recent recommendations by the Canadian Hypertension Society, the National Kidney Foundation and the American Diabetes Association, strongly suggest that to maximally preserve renal function and reduce cardiovascular morbidity and mortality, a blood pressure goal <130/80 mmHg is required.[14–16] Therefore, it is proposed that in diabetic patients with hypertension and/or renal impairment, the blood pressure goal should be 130/80 mmHg. Additionally, for diabetic patients with proteinuria of >1 g per day, the optimal blood pressure goal should be 125/75 mmHg.[13]

An important issue is whether more aggressive lowering of blood pressure poses any risk along with these demonstrated benefits. Excessive blood pressure lowering could lead to acute cardiac or neurological complications, nullifying the long-term cardiovascular benefit. Earlier retrospective studies suggested the possibility of a J-shaped curve with regard to cardiovascular events and level of blood pressure reduction.[21,22] However, in clinical trials published over the past 5 years,

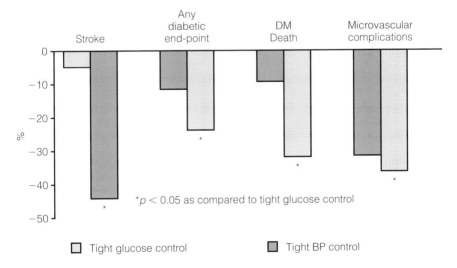

Figure 3.2

Rate of cardiovascular risk reduction of tight blood pressure (BP) control versus tight glucose control. DM, diabetes mellitus.

randomized patients with type 2 diabetes and hypertension who achieve levels of diastolic blood pressure reduction to <85 mmHg, show no significant increase in the rate of adverse cardiovascular or renal events.[23] Indeed, in the HOT and UKPDS 38 trials, the groups randomized to the lowest level of blood pressure control – especially the diabetic cohort – had the greatest reduction in cardiovascular events.

Choice of drug therapy

A review of clinical trials that randomized patients with either diabetes or renal impairment to two different levels of blood pressure reduction demonstrated that those randomized to the lower level of blood pressure required an average of 3.2 different antihypertensive medications to be taken daily (*Fig. 3.3*).[15] These lower blood pressure groups had much lower cardiovascular event rates and slower progression of renal disease compared to the higher blood pressure groups.

ACE inhibitors

All international and national recommendations, including those of the JNC VI and the World Health Organization (WHO), provide a logical approach to the use of antihypertensive drug therapy in diabetics.[13,24,25] The JNC VI recommend ACE inhibitors as the preferred initial therapy in diabetic patients with blood pressures >130/85 mmHg. It is well known

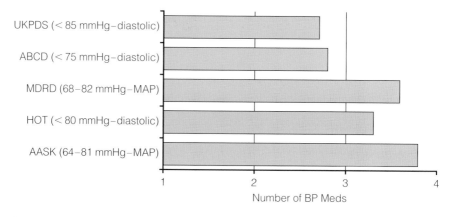

Figure 3.3

Average number of different blood pressure medications (BP Meds) taken daily to achieve desired goal blood pressure in trials that randomized for different levels of blood pressure control.

that ACE inhibitors prevent or delay progression of diabetic nephropathy to a degree that surpasses that expected from blood pressure lowering alone. In fact, in a meta-analysis by Weidman *et al*,[26] ACE inhibitors reduced proteinuria in diabetic patients without lowering blood pressure.

Additionally, the recent results of the Heart Outcomes Prevention Evaluation (HOPE) trial clearly demonstrate the benefit of ACE inhibitors in diabetic patients. In this trial, 9297 patients with vascular disease or diabetes and one other cardiovascular risk factor were randomly assigned to a once-daily ACE inhibitor at maximal dose or placebo. The primary outcomes were a composite of myocardial infarction, stroke or cardiovascular death. The results indicate that treatment with ACE inhibitors reduced the rates of myocardial infarction by 80%, stroke by 68% and cardiovascular death by 74%.[27] Furthermore, in the MIcroalbuminuria, Cardiovascular, and Renal Outcomes substudy of the HOPE (MICRO-HOPE) trial, 3577 people with diabetes included in the study, who had had a previous cardiovascular event or had at least one other cardiovascular risk factor, and had no clinical proteinuria, heart failure, or low ejection fraction, and were not taking ACE inhibitors, were randomly assigned to ramipril (10 mg daily) or placebo. The primary outcome was development of overt nephropathy. This study noted a 24% relative risk reduction of overt nephropathy in the intervention group after 4.5 years of follow-up, an effect independent of blood pressure reduction.[28]

Initiating therapy with ACE inhibitors may lead to an elevation in serum creatinine. This should not lead to discontinuation, since an analysis of renal trials that measured early and late changes in glomerular filtration rate showed that increases in serum creatinine limited up to 30% above a baseline up to 3 mg daily, within the first 4 months of starting an ACE inhibitor correlated with slower rates of decline in renal function after 3 years or more of follow-up. Additionally, long-term rates of decline in renal function were closer in individuals who achieved pressure values of $\leqslant 130/80$ mmHg.[9]

Angiotensin II-receptor blockers (ARB)

These agents are the most recent and best tolerated of all antihypertensive drug classes, with an apparent beneficial profile similar to ACE inhibitors. Preliminary studies indicate that ARB may have reno- and cardioprotective effects to at least the same degree as those provided by ACE inhibitors. For the kidney, the conclusion of two large trials involving >3000 people with nephropathy associated with type 2 diabetes solidifies the role of this class as renoprotective agents. The Irebesartan Diabetic Nephropathy Trial (IDNT)[29] and the Reduction of Endpoints in NIDDM with the AII Antagonist Losartan (RENAAL) trial[30] both demonstrated a 22% risk reduction of renal disease progression compared to comparable blood pressure control achieved with conventional therapy.

Moreover, the IDNT trial confirmed previous reports suggesting that dihydropyridine CCB do not protect against renal disease progression as well as ARB, since they increased the risk of renal disease progression by 7% in the IDNT trial.

ARB may have another advantage over ACE inhibitors; they have less associated hyperkalemia. A recent multicentred, randomized crossover study showed that people with an average glomerular filtration rate (GFR) of 44 ml per minute had a significantly smaller increase in serum potassium and less hyperkalemia while on ARB compared to those randomized to an ACE inhibitor, further confirming the concept that ARB have fewer adverse effects than ACE inhibitors.[31] Thus, from the standpoint of the kidney, the data currently suggest that ARB not only protect against progression but also are better tolerated than ACE inhibitors.

Diuretics

Additional antihypertensive agent(s) may subsequently be added to the ACE inhibitor as needed to achieve the goal blood pressure. In many patients with diabetes as well as with normal or slightly reduced renal function, addition of low-dose thiazide diuretics, i.e. 12–25 mg per day, offer an augmented benefit to achieve the target blood pressure goal. These agents have additive blood-pressure-reducing effects, especially in African-Americans, and have also been shown to reduce cardiovascular events.[32]

CCB

The renoprotective effects and additional benefits of CCB are less uniform. There have been no definitive trials of renal disease progression with CCB except for two recent studies: the IDNT in diabetic nephropathy[29] and the African-American Study of Kidney Disease and Hypertension (AASK) trial in non-diabetic renal disease.[33] These trials both show that dihydropyridine CCB should not be used to lower blood pressure in the absence of an ACE inhibitor or an ARB, since they do not reduce the rate of renal disease progression in spite of blood pressure reduction. The cardiovascular effects of these agents are also less clear; while they clearly protect against stokes, recent trials, including the Fosinopril Amlodipine Cardiac Events Trial (FACET)[34], and the Appropriate Blood Pressure Control in Diabetes (ABCD) trial,[35] have demonstrated a failure to reduce cardiovascular risk. A recent meta-analysis by MacMahon and colleagues[36] demonstrates that CCB are not harmful.[36] In FACET, the best results were obtained when CCB and ACE inhibitors were given concomitantly, although the results were not statistically different from those who received the ACE inhibitor alone. Moreover, the group that received combination therapy also had significantly lower blood pressures compared to the other groups. Conversely, in the diabetes subgroup of HOT and the Syst-Eur trial,[37] a long-acting dihydropyridine calcium antagonist significantly reduced cardiovascular events. In both of these trials, this reduction in events was primarily driven by stroke reduction and many of these patients were receiving ACE inhibitors concomitantly, 73% in the HOT trial and 43% in the Syst-Eur trial. To date, none of the dihydropyridine CCB currently available in the USA has been shown to reduce ischemic cardiovascular events in randomized secondary prevention trials of survivors of acute myocardial infarction when used in the absence of an ACE inhibitor or a β-blocker.[8,38]

β-blockers

In patients with diabetes, β-blockers reduce cardiovascular risk in spite of their adverse metabolic effects.[39] However, cavedilol is currently the only β-blocker that has demonstrated cardiovascular risk reduction with neutral metabolic effects.[40] Also, β-blockers have additive blood-pressure-lowering effects to most antihypertensive agents in patients with baseline pulse rates >84 beats per minute.[41] At pulse rates <84 beats per minute there is little effect on blood pressure when β-blockers are combined with ACE inhibitors.

α-blockers

Other classes of antihypertensive agents, such as α-blockers, are effective in lowering blood pressure and are associated with favorable metabolic profiles in patients with diabetes.[42] However, in the Antihypertensive and Lipid Lowering treatment to prevent Heart Attack Trial (ALLHAT), the α-blocker doxazosin treatment arm was discontinued because of a higher incidence of congestive heart failure and less benefit in preventing ischemic heart disease compared to the diuretic chlorthalidone.[43] Given these data, α-blockers should not be used as initial therapy but they may be useful as adjunctive therapy to help achieve the blood pressure goal, especially in older men when used with prostatism.

Combination antihypertensive medications

The use of combination antihypertensive medications, such as an ACE inhibitor combined with either a diuretic or a calcium antagonist, may be useful to reduce pill counts and may also improve patient adherence. These combinations achieve blood pressure goals in >80% of diabetic patients with hypertension,[19] thus resulting in a more consistent and cost-effective control of hypertension.[44]

Suggested approach to achieve blood pressure goals in diabetes

Based on data that evaluate achievement of blood pressure goals in the setting of an outpatient general medicine clinic, it is apparent that if systolic blood pressure and/or diastolic blood pressure is 15 or 10 mmHg above the desired blood pressure goal, respectively, then at least two different antihypertensive agents would be needed to achieve the desired goal.[15] Thus, if the goal blood pressure is 130/80 mmHg, the patient has a clinic reading >145/90 mmHg and is not receiving treatment, the physician will need to prescribe two different agents to achieve the goal blood pressure. These data, taken together with the results of clinical trials in cardiovascular and renal disease, have led to the following paradigm to achieve the recommended blood pressure goal for patients with diabetes with or without renal insufficiency (Fig. 3.4). It should be noted that the suggested paradigm applies only to patients who have diabetes or renal insufficiency but without other co-morbid conditions such as angina or heart failure, or immediately following myocar-

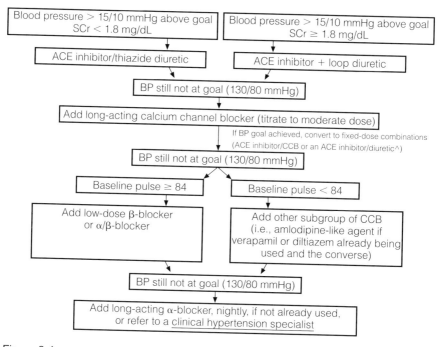

Figure 3.4

Suggested approach for achieving blood pressure (BP) goals in patients with diabetes and or renal insufficiency. Scr, serum creatinine. Reprinted with permission from Bakris et al.[15]

dial infarction. ACE inhibitor/diuretic combinations are ideal as initial therapy to achieve the blood pressure goal of 130/80 mmHg. Diuretics potentiate the blood-pressure-lowering effects of ACE inhibitors, especially in African-Americans and the elderly. If ACE inhibitors are not tolerated, ARB may be substituted. CCB are meaningful second-line agents because they demonstrate an additive blood-pressure-lowering capability when used with either ACE inhibitors or diuretics. Moreover, when ACE inhibitors are used in concert with CCB they have resulted in reduction of cardiovascular events.[19,34] Conversely, combinations of β-blockers and ACE inhibitors have failed to show any additive benefit on blood pressure reduction if the baseline pulse rate is <84 beats per minute.[41] Thus, β-blockers may provide additional blood pressure reduction only in patients whose pulse rates are >84 beats per minute and not at goal blood pressure. Other agents such as hydralazine or minoxidil, and clinidine or methyldopa can be used as adjunctive therapy to help achieve goal blood pressure.

Conclusions

A review of the currently available evidence indicates that in patients with diabetes and/or renal insufficiency, the goal blood pressure should be 130/80 mmHg. Lower blood pressure levels, i.e.<125/75 mmHg, are recommended for people who have proteinuria >1 g per day and renal insufficiency regardless of etiology. At the lower blood pressure goal there is also superior benefit than with conventional blood pressure goal for reduction of cardiovascular risk in patients with diabetes, whether they have pre-existing renal disease or not. It is clear that control of blood pressure to the revised lower goal is of utmost importance for improving both cardiovascular and renal outcomes in patients with diabetes. Antihypertensive regimes should include ACE inhibitors in order to provide maximum cardio- and renoprotection in these patients. Data from several major recent prospective trials, including UKPDS 38 and HOT trials, demonstrate, however, that attainment of this lower blood pressure goal is virtually impossible with monotherapy. The majority of the time addition of multiple antihypertensive medications including diuretics, CCB or any similar combination is required to achieve this lower blood pressure goal. Physicians must make every effort to achieve the blood pressure goal by the least intrusive means possible. This will minimize drug-related side effects, improve patient adherence, and reduce cardiovascular and renal events.

References

1. Nelson RG, Knowler WC, Pettit DJ, Bennett PH. Kidney disease in diabetes. Diabetes in America, National Institutes of Health Publication No 95-1468 (2nd edn) 1995, 349–400.

2. Rachmani R, Ravid M. Risk factors for nephropathy in type 2 diabetes mellitus. Compr Ther 1999; 2: 366–369.

3. Mogensen CE, Hansen KW, Pedersen MM, Christensen CK. Renal factors influencing blood pressure threshold and choice of treatment for hypertension in IDDM. Diabetes Care 1991; 14 (suppl 4): 13–26.

4. US Renal Data System (USRDS) Annual Data Report. National Institutes of Health, National Institute of Diabetes & Digestive Kidney Diseases. Bethesda, MD, April 1999.

5. Haffner SM, Lehto S, Ronnernaa T et al. Mortality from coronary heart disease in subjects with type 2 diabetes and in nondiabetic subjects with and without prior myocardial infarction. N Engl J Med 1998; 339: 229–234.

6. Peterson JC, Adler S, Burkart JM et al. Blood pressure control, proteinuria, and the progression of renal disease. The Modification of Diet in Renal Disease Study. Ann Intern Med 1995; 123: 754–762.

7. Ravid M, Lang R, Rachmani R, Lishner M. Long-term renoprotective effect of angiotensin-converting enzyme inhibition in non-insulin-dependent diabetes mellitus. A 7-year follow-up study. Arch Intern Med 1996; 156: 286–289.

8. Sheinfeld GR, Bakris GL. Benefits of combination angiotensin-converting enzyme inhibitor and calcium antagonist therapy for diabetic patients. Am J Hypertens 1999; 12: 80S–85S.

9. Bakris GL, Weir MR. ACE inhibitor-associated elevations in serum creatinine: is this a cause for concern? Arch Intern Med 2000; 160: 685–693.

10. Keane WF, Eknoyan G. Proteinuria, Albuminuria, Risk Assessment, Detection, Elimination (PARADE): a position paper of the National Kidney Foundation. Am J Kidney Dis 1999; 33: 1004–1010.

11. Tuttle KR, Puhlman ME, Cooney SK, Short R. Urinary albumin and insulin as predictors of coronary artery disease: an angiographic study. Am J Kidney Dis 1999; 34: 918–925.

12. Bakris GL, Weir MR, DeQuattro V, McMahon FG. Effects of an ACE inhibitor/calcium antagonist combination on proteinuria in diabetic nephropathy. Kidney Int 1998; 54: 1283–1289.

13. Joint National Committee on Detection, Evaluation, and Treatment of High Blood Pressure. The sixth report of the Joint National Committee on Detection, Evaluation, and Treatment of High Blood Pressure (JNC VI). Arch Intern Med 1997; 154: 2413–2446.

14. Feldman RD. The 1999 Canadian recommendations for the management of hypertension. On behalf of the Task Force for the Development of the 1999 Canadian Recommendations for the Management of Hypertension. Can J Cardiol 1999; 15 (suppl G): 57G–64G.

15. Bakris GL, Williams M, Dworkin L et al. Preserving renal function in adults with hypertension and diabetes: a consensus approach. National Kidney Foundation Hypertension and Diabetes executive Committees working group.

Am J Kidney Dis 2000; 36: 646–661.

16. American Diabetes Association Clinical Practice Recommendations 2001. Diabetes Care 2001; 24: S1–S133.

17. Bakris GL. Maximizing cardiorenal benefits: achieve blood pressure goals. J Clin Hypertens 1999; 1: 141–148.

18. Lazarus JM, Bourgoignie JJ, Buckalew VM *et al.* Achievement and safety of a low BP goal in chronic renal disease. The Modification of Diet in Renal Disease Study Group. Hypertension 1997; 29: 641–650.

19. Hansson L, Zanchetti A, Carruthers SG *et al.* Effects of intensive blood pressure lowering and low-dose aspirin in patients with hypertension: principal results of the Hypertension Optimal Treatment (HOT) randomised trial. The HOT Study Group. Lancet 1998; 351: 1755–1762.

20. Tight blood pressure control and risk of macrovascular and microvascular complications in type 2 diabetes: UKPDS 38. UK Prospective Diabetes Study Group. BMJ 1998; 317: 703–713.

21. Cruickshank JM, Thorp JM, Zacharias FJ. Benefits and potential harm of lowering high blood pressure. Lancet 1987; 1: 581–584.

22. Farnett L, Mulrow CD, Linn WD *et al.* The J-curve phenomenon and the treatment of hypertension. Is there a point beyond which pressure reduction is dangerous? JAMA 1991; 265: 489–495.

23. Kaplan N. J-curve not burned off by HOT study. Hypertension Optimal Treatment (comment). Lancet 1998; 351: 1748–1749.

24. American Diabetes Association. Clinical Practice Recommendations 1999. Diabetes Care 1999; 22 (suppl 1): S1–S114.

25. Chalmers J, MacMahon S, Mancia G *et al.* World Health Organization–International Society of Hypertension Guidelines for the Management of Hypertension. Guidelines sub-committee. Clin Exp Hypertens 1999; 21: 1009–1060.

26. Weidmann P, Schneider M, Bohlen L. Therapeutic efficacy of different antihypertensive drugs on human diabetic nephropathy: an updated meta-analysis. Nephrol Dial Transplant 1995; 10 (suppl 9): 39–45.

27. The Heart Outcomes Prevention Evaluation Study Investigators. Effects of an angiotensin-converting-enzyme inhibitor, ramipril, on cardiovascular events in high-risk patients. N Engl J Med 2000; 342: 145–153.

28. Lewis EJ, Hunsicker LG, Clarke WR *et al.* Renoprotective effect of the angiotensin-receptor antagonist irbesartan in patients with nephropathy due to type 2 diabetes. N Engl J Med 2001; 345: 851–860.

29. Brenner BM, Cooper ME, de Zeeuw D *et al.* Effects of losartan on renal and cardiovascular outcomes in patients with type 2 diabetes and nephropathy. N Engl J Med 2001; 345: 861–869.

30. Heart Outcomes Prevention Evaluation (HOPE) Study Investigators. Effects of ramipril on cardiovascular and microvascular outcomes in people with diabetes mellitus: results of the HOPE study and MICRO-HOPE substudy. Lancet 2000; 355: 253–259.

31. Bakris GL, Siomos M, Richardson D *et al.* ACE inhibition or angiotensin receptor blocker-impact on potassium in renal failure. VAL-K study group. Kidney Int 2000; 58: 2084–2092.

32. Epstein M, Bakris GL. Newer approaches to antihypertensive

therapy: use of fixed-dose combination therapy. Arch Intern Med 1996; 156: 1969–1978.

33. Tatti P, Pahor M, Byington RP *et al.* Outcome results of the Fosinopril versus Amlodipine Cardiovascular Events randomized Trial (FACET) in patients with hypertension and NIDDM. Diabetes Care 1998; 21: 597–610.

34. Agodoa LY, Appel L, Bakris GL *et al.* African-American Study of Kidney Disease and Hypertension (AASK) Study Group: effect of ramipril vs amlodipine on renal outcomes in hypertensive nephrosclerosis: a randomized controlled trial. JAMA 2001; 285: 2774–2728.

35. Estacio RO, Barrett JW, Hiatt WR *et al.* The effect of nisoldipine as compared with enalapril on cardiovascular outcomes in patients with non-insulin-dependent diabetes and hypertension. N Engl J Med 1998; 338: 645–652.

36. Neal B, MacMahon S, Chapman N. Effects of ACE inhibitors, calcium antagonists, and other blood pressure lowering drugs: results of prospectively designed overviews of randomized trials. Blood Pressure Lowering Treatment Trialists' Collaboration. Lancet 2000; 356: 1955–1964.

37. Tuomilehto J, Rastenyte D, Birkenhager WH *et al.* Effects of calcium-channel blockade in older patients with diabetes and systolic hypertension. Systolic Hypertension in Europe Trial Investigators. N Engl J Med 1999; 340: 677–684.

38. Packer M, O'Connor CM, Ghali JK *et al.* Effect of amlodipine on morbidity and mortality in severe chronic heart failure. Prospective Randomized Amlodipine Survival Evaluation Study Group. N Engl J Med 1996; 335: 1107–1114.

39. Gress TW, Nieto FJ, Shahar E *et al.* for the Atherosclerosis Risk in Communities Study. Hypertension and antihypertensive therapy and the risk factors for the type 2 diabetes mellitus. N Engl J Med 2000; 342: 905–912.

40. Giugliano D, Acampora R, Marfella R *et al.* Metabolic and cardiovascular effects of carvedilol and atenolol in non-insulin-dependent diabetes mellitus and hypertension. A randomized, controlled trial. Ann Intern Med 1997; 126: 955–959.

41. Belz GG, Breithaupt K, Erb K *et al.* Influence of the angiotensin converting enzyme inhibitor cilazapril, the beta-blocker propranolol and their combination on haemodynamics in hypertension. J Hypertens 1989; 7: 817–824.

42. Giordano M, Matsuda M, Sanders L *et al.* Effects of angiotensin-converting enzyme inhibitors, calcium channel antagonists, and alpha-adrenergic blockers on glucose and lipid metabolism in non-insulin-dependent diabetes mellitus patients with hypertension. Diabetes 1995; 44: 665–671.

43. ALLHAT. Collaborative Research Group. Major cardiovascular events in hypertensive patients randomized to doxazosin vs clorthalidone: the antihypertensive and lipid-lowering treatment to prevent heart attack trial (ALLHAT). JAMA 2000; 283: 2013–2014.

44. Elliott WJ, Weir DR, Black HR. Cost-effectiveness of the new lower blood pressure goal of JNC VI for diabetic hypertensives. Arch Intern Med 2000; 160: 1277–1283.

45. Ifudu O. Benefits of combination antihypertensive therapy in progressive chronic renal failure. Am J Managed Care 1999; 5 (suppl II): 429S–448S.

4
The roles of sodium, potassium and calcium in the treatment of hypertension

Paul Muntner, Jiang He and Paul K Whelton

Introduction

Clinical trials have demonstrated that lifestyle modification offers the potential for lowering blood pressure and the concomitant risk of cardiovascular disease with minimal adverse effects on the patient. Therefore, lifestyle modifications have generally been recommended as a means to prevent hypertension and as an initial approach in treating stage 1 and 2 hypertension in persons without target-organ damage and cardiovascular disease.[1-3] Lifestyle modification interventions that have been proven to be efficacious include weight loss, increased physical activity, alteration in dietary macronutrient intake, reduced alcohol consumption, reduced sodium intake and potassium supplementation.[3,4] The purpose of this chapter is to provide an overview, including the most recent available evidence, on the role of sodium reduction and potassium and calcium supplementation in the treatment of hypertension.

Dietary intake of sodium, potassium and calcium are highly correlated. However, because much of the evidence regarding the role of these factors in modulating levels of blood pressure has been assessed autonomously (e.g. calcium supplementation trials have kept participant's sodium and potassium intake unaltered) each factor will be discussed separately. Recent clinical trial experience pertaining to sodium reduction in the context of a diet high in fruit, vegetables and low-fat dairy products will be discussed at the end of this chapter.

Sodium reduction

Dietary sodium was first implicated in the etiology and pathogenesis of hypertension early in the twentieth century.[5] In the 1940s, Kempner[6] reported that a low-sodium rice diet resulted in a substantial reduction in blood pressure among a sizable proportion of persons with severe hypertension. In 1960, Dahl[7] showed that dietary sodium intake was a major determinant of blood pressure across human populations. Evidence from animal experiments,[8-11] observational studies[12] and randomized controlled trials[13-17] published over the past several decades have yielded a large body of evidence that reduction of dietary sodium intake lowers blood pressure.

Animal experiments

In the 1940s, the first animal study underscored the role of high salt intake in the causation of elevated blood pressure. Subsequently, thousands of animal experiments investigating the role of dietary sodium on blood pressure have been conducted. Most of these studies have been carried out in rats, providing important data but with limited applicability to humans.[11,18] In 1995, Denton *et al.*[11] reported on a seminal experimental study in which 26 chimpanzees were fed either a diet low in sodium or sequentially a diet low in sodium for 1 year, high in sodium for 1 year and, finally, low in sodium for the remaining weeks of the 2.5-year study period. While the chimpanzees on the low-sodium diet experienced no significant change in blood pressure during follow-up, those receiving salt supplementation experienced a rise in systolic and diastolic blood pressure of 33 and 10 mmHg (each $p < 0.01$), respectively (*Fig. 4.1*). Upon returning to a low-salt diet, their blood pressure fell to its baseline level. This and other experimental data unequivocally demonstrate that dietary salt intake has a direct effect on blood pressure in animals.

Observational evidence

The study of dietary sodium intake on blood pressure within populations has been limited by a number of methodological challenges,[19] including variation in an individual's day-to-day sodium intake,[9] the relatively narrow distribution of sodium intake within populations[20,21] and the wide variability of blood pressure values at the same level of sodium intake.[22-24] Further complicating the interpretation of this relationship is the influence and interaction of environmental exposures and genetic factors on blood pressure, and the use of different methods to assess sodium intake.[25] Some studies have used dietary recall to assess sodium intake while others have used 24-hour urinary sodium excretion.[21] The strengths and weaknesses of each of these methods have been previously noted.[26-29] Due to these limitations, much of the observational evidence documenting the benefit of a reduced sodium intake has been derived from across population studies.[21]

In 1960, Dahl[7] reported a strong positive association between average sodium intake and mean blood pressure across five geographically diverse populations. Several subsequent studies have confirmed this association.[30-32] The most important observational study of the association

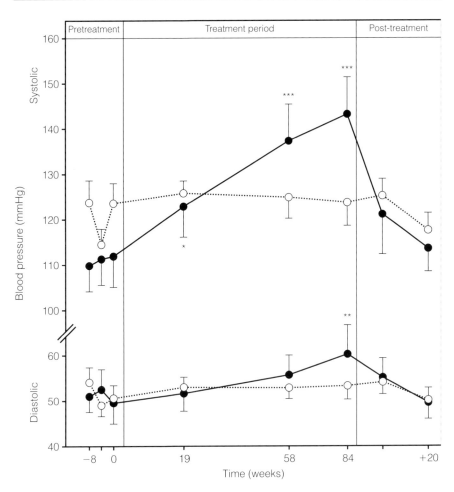

Figure 4.1

Mean systolic and diastolic blood pressures in 10 experimental chimpanzees (●) and 12 control animals (○) during three phases (pretreatment, treatment, post-treatment). Dietary salt was added progressively to the diet of the experimental group during the treatment period. Modified from Denton et al.[11]

between sodium intake and blood pressure is the INTERSALT study.[20] The INTERSALT study was a cross-sectional investigation among 10,079 men and women between the ages of 20 and 59 from 52 populations within 32 countries.[33] Blood pressure and a single estimate of 24-hour urinary sodium were obtained by trained observers using a standardized protocol. In cross-population analysis, a 100 mmol per 24 hour lower level of urinary excretion of sodium was associated with a 7.1 and 3.8 mmHg lower level of systolic and diastolic blood pressure, respectively. After further standardization for median prevalence of alcohol drinking, amount of alcohol intake among drinkers and body mass index (BMI), systolic and diastolic blood pressures were 4.5 and 2.3 mmHg lower for a 100 mmol lower level of urinary sodium excretion.

There are limitations to inferences derived from across population studies.[34,35] First, it is difficult to collect data from such studies in a standardized manner.[30] Additionally, the correlation detected may reflect the effect of an unmeasured confounding variable.[21] Also, the potential for ecological fallacy is present; it is not known whether individuals with the high dietary sodium intake are also those with a higher blood pressure.[35,36] Evidence from the INTERSALT study is, however, not limited to cross-population analysis. In a pooled within-population analysis of INTERSALT, those with a 100 mmol per day lower level of 24-hour urinary sodium excretion had a 4.3 and 1.8 mmHg lower level of systolic and diastolic blood pressure, respectively.[37] Although these data do not provide definitive proof of causality, they offer strong suggestive evidence for such a relationship and an impetus for further investigation of the effectiveness of sodium reduction in the treatment of hypertension.

Clinical trials of sodium reduction

Randomized controlled trials are considered to be the gold standard for measuring the efficacy of an intervention. Therefore, despite the impressive results from observational studies, evidence from clinical trials that reduced sodium intake lowers blood pressure is necessary prior to recommending it as a means to treat hypertension.

Several recent clinical trials have provided evidence that a moderate reduction in sodium intake substantially reduces blood pressure.[38–40] In the Trial of Non-pharmacologic Interventions in the Elderly, conducted in 875 participants between the ages of 60 and 80 with well-controlled hypertension, mean systolic and diastolic blood pressure reductions were greater in those randomized to sodium reduction compared to their counterparts randomized to usual care (*Table 4.1*). Also, the percentage of persons who were able to discontinue antihypertensive medication and remain drug free while maintaining their blood pressure below 150/90 mmHg, and remaining free of a hypertension-related clinical complication, was significantly higher among those assigned to a sodium reduction group compared to their counterparts assigned to usual care (38 versus 24%, $p < 0.001$). Meta-analysis of randomized clinical trials provides a means to formally pool and quantify findings from several clinical trials in a standardized and objective manner. Cutler *et al.*[16] performed a meta-analysis using all randomized controlled trials reported throughout January 1990. Among the 18 trials conducted in patients with hypertension, both systolic and diastolic blood pressures were significantly reduced (*Table 4.1*). Even larger reductions in blood pressure

Table 4.1 Effect and 95% confidence interval (CI) of sodium reduction on systolic and diastolic blood pressures from one large clinical trial and from two meta-analysis studies of persons with hypertension

Study	Systolic blood pressure (mmHg)	Diastolic blood pressure (mmHg)
Trials of Nonpharmacologic Interventions in the Elderly	−2.6 (−4.8, −0.4)	−1.1 (−2.5, 0.3)
Meta-analysis* (Cutler et al.)[16]	−4.9 (−6.2, −3.7)	−2.6 (−4.3, −1.0)
Meta-analysis* (Midgley et al.)[18,41]	−5.9 (−7.8, −4.1)	−3.8 (−4.8, −2.9)

*Results presented are limited to participants with hypertension.

were demonstrated in a subsequent meta-analysis using 28 clinical trials conducted in hypertensive patients.[18,41] No safety concerns were reported in the reduced sodium diet.

Sodium intake and cardiovascular disease outcomes

Several ecological studies have identified a positive relationship between average population dietary sodium intake and mortality due to cardiovascular disease (CVD) and stroke. However, data from prospective intrapopulation studies are limited. Two studies have been conducted using data from the First National Health and Nutrition Examination Survey (NHANES I) Epidemiological Follow-up study, a representative sample of the US population that has been actively followed for 17–21 years.[42,43] Although using the same data, these studies reached different conclusions. One study (Alderman et al.)[43] did not find an association between higher sodium intake and an increase in CVD mortality; however, a subsequent study (He et al.)[42] found a significant increased risk of mortality from stroke, CVD, coronary heart disease (CHD), and all causes among overweight participants (Fig. 4.2). In the latter study, among overweight adults, for each 100 mmol higher sodium intake per 24 hours, the risk increased by 89% for stroke, 44% for CHD, 61% for CVD and 39% for all causes (each $p \leqslant 0.02$). Differences in the results between these two studies may have resulted from differences in the hypotheses explored, exclusion criteria, analysis methodology, and the interaction between being overweight and the effect of sodium on blood pressure.

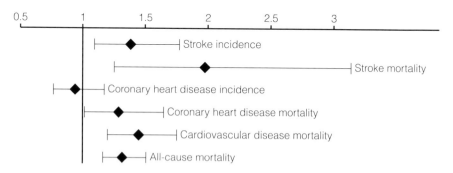

Figure 4.2

Relative risk of stroke incidence and mortality, coronary heart disease (CHD) incidence and mortality, cardiovascular disease (CVD) mortality and all-cause mortality associated with 50 mmol per day higher dietary sodium intake among 2688 overweight participants in the NHANES I Epidemiological Follow-up study during 17–21 years of follow-up. From He et al.[42]

In summary, moderate reduction of dietary sodium intake results in a substantial decrease in blood pressure. Both the American Heart Association and the National Health Lung and Blood Institute advocate limiting dietary sodium to no more than 100 mmol per day. It has been estimated that reducing dietary sodium intake to this level, in Western populations, would result in a 6% lower risk of stroke and a 4% lower risk of ischemic heart disease.[44] Although, the response may vary by subpopulation, sodium reduction could substantially reduce the societal burden of CVD morbidity and mortality.

Potassium supplementation

The first clinical trial of potassium supplementation was reported in 1928.[45] Although evidence from animal studies has consistently supported the hypothesis that potassium supplementation lowers blood pressure,[46-48] evidence from humans has proven less consistent.[25,49] In part, this is because the largest and most rigorously designed trials of potassium supplementation have yielded the least impressive results.[50] Although still controversial, the balance of evidence supports the role of potassium supplementation in lowering blood pressure and is recommended by the sixth Joint National Committee on the detection, evaluation, and treatment of hypertension (JNC VI).[3]

Animal experiments

Evidence has been collected in animals regarding the effects of both potassium depletion[51-53] and supplementation.[54,55] The presence and magnitude of a rise in blood pressure after potassium depletion has been variable depending on the animal model and the method of potassium administration. In contrast, potassium supplementation has lowered blood pressure in several experimental models, including salt-sensitive Dahl rats, Wistar rats with two-kidney and one-clip renovascular hypertension, and dog models. Proposed mechanisms include a reduction in exchangeable sodium content and a reduced peripheral vascular resistance.[56,57] Overall, potassium supplementation has consistently been shown to lower blood pressure in experimental models of hypertension.[46-48]

Observational evidence

Both interpopulation[58] and within-population[59,60] studies have provided evidence of a relationship between dietary potassium intake and level of blood pressure. In the INTERSALT study, after adjustment for age, sex, BMI, alcohol consumption and urinary sodium excretion, a difference in urinary potassium excretion of 50 mmol per day was associated with 3.36 and 1.87 mmHg lower systolic and diastolic blood pressure level, respectively, across the 52 study populations.[58] Among the several within-population studies yielding information on the relationship between dietary potassium intake and blood pressure,[61–63] Watson et al.[64] found a significant negative correlation between diastolic blood pressure and 24-hour urinary potassium excretion. Additionally, an inverse correlation was present between 24-hour urinary potassium excretion and systolic blood pressure, and a positive correlation between the sodium/potassium ratio among 662 adolescent girls in Mississippi.

Prospective studies have provided marginal evidence of an inverse relationship between potassium intake and the incidence of hypertension. Among 58,218 predominantly white women in the Nurses Health Study, those with a potassium intake >3200 mg per day had a relative risk of incident hypertension over 4 years of follow-up of 0.77 compared to their counterparts with an intake <2000 mg per day ($p < 0.001$) after adjustment for age, BMI and alcohol consumption.[65] However, the relative risk was 1.05 and non-significant after further adjustment for dietary intake of fiber, calcium and magnesium. In the Health Professionals Follow-up Study, the relationship between dietary potassium intake and incident hypertension was investigated among 30,681 men between the ages of 40 and 75.[66] After adjustment for age, BMI and alcohol intake, men with a potassium intake ⩾3600 mg per day had a significantly lower risk of hypertension compared to those with an intake <2400 mg per day ($p < 0.01$). After further adjustment for dietary intake of calcium, magnesium and fiber, the relative risk was 0.83 but was no longer significant. Because of the high correlation between potassium intake and other dietary variables, observational studies provide only limited capacity to make causal inferences.

Clinical trials of potassium supplementation

Since the first report of the benefit of potassium supplementation in lowering blood pressure in 1928, over 60 clinical trials have been published.[67,68] Many of these trials have been small and underpowered. However, several meta-analyses of the randomized controlled trials of potassium supplementation have yielded evidence that potassium supplementation lowers blood pressure. In the largest and most recent of these, published in 1997 by Whelton et al.,[67] 33 randomized clinical trials that met prespecified inclusion requirements were analyzed.[67] One of these trials was an outlier and reported an extreme reduction in systolic and diastolic blood pressure in the potassium supplementation group of 41 and 17 mmHg, respectively. Even after exclusion of this trial, however, potassium supplementation was associated with a significant reduction in mean [95% confidence interval (CI)] systolic and diastolic blood pressures of 3.11 (1.91, 4.31) and 1.97 mmHg (0.52, 3.42), respectively. Treatment-related declines in systolic blood pressure were significantly greater for the six trials with >80% black participants compared to the 25 trials with >80% white participants ($p = 0.03$; *Fig. 4.3*). The reduction in systolic and diastolic blood pressure among those receiving potassium supplementation was also larger at higher levels of sodium intake. A majority of the clinical trials excluded from this meta-analysis provided results that were consistent with the hypothesis that potassium administration reduces blood pressure. Most clinical trials' experience to date emanates from studies in which potassium was administered in pill form as a chloride salt; however, there is little reason to suspect different outcomes depending on whether potassium is administered as a dietary supplement, as non-chloride salt or by increased fruit and vegetable intake.

Potassium intake and CVD events

Ecological studies, including INTERSALT, have identified the presence of an inverse relationship between potassium intake and stroke mortality, and a positive relationship between the sodium/potassium ratio and stroke mortality.[69,70] Additionally, several within-population studies have indicated that high-potassium diets are protective against stroke and kidney disease.[71,72] In a study of 859 persons in a retirement village who were followed for 12 years, Khaw and Barrett-Connor[73] reported that dietary potassium intake was protective against stroke incidence.[73] Specifically, a 10 mmol higher level of dietary potassium intake was

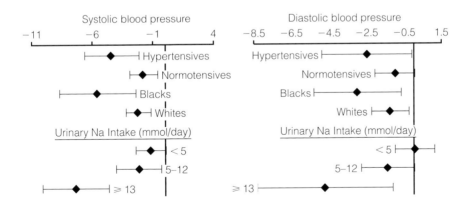

Figure 4.3

Reduction in systolic and diastolic blood pressures comparing persons receiving potassium supplementation to their counterparts receiving placebo from 32 randomized controlled trials by subgroup. Modified from Whelton *et al*.[67]

associated with a relative risk (95% CI) of stroke of 0.60 (0.44, 0.82) after adjustment for sex, age, systolic blood pressure, serum total cholesterol, fasting plasma glucose, BMI and current smoking. In the much larger and more representative NHANES Epidemiologic Follow-up study, 927 stroke events occurred over an average of 19 years of follow-up.[74] In age and energy adjusted analyses, Bazzano et al.[74] noted that persons consuming <34.6 mmol potassium per day had a 37% (relative risk = 1.37; 95% CI: 1.20, 1.54; $p < 0.001$) higher hazard of stroke than their counterparts who were consuming more potassium per day. The relative hazards estimate was not substantially altered by additional adjustment for established CVD risk factors and dietary factors. After adjustment for age, race, sex, systolic blood pressure, serum cholesterol, BMI, history of diabetes, physical activity, education level, regular alcohol consumption, current cigarette smoking, vitamin supplement use and other dietary factors, persons consuming <34.6 mmol potassium per day experienced a 28% higher hazard of stroke than their counterparts consuming more potassium (Table 4.2).

In summary, evidence from clinical trials of potassium supplementation is consistent and supports the beneficial effects on blood pressure. Current JNC VI guidelines recommend 'an adequate intake of potassium (approximately 90-mmol per day), preferably from food sources such as fresh fruits and vegetables, should be maintained'.[3]

Calcium supplementation

The hypothesis of an inverse relationship between dietary calcium and blood pressure stemmed from reports in the 1960s relating hard drinking water to lower mortality from CVD.[75,77] Since these early reports, experi-

Table 4.2   Hazard ratio and 95% confidence interval (CI) of stroke mortality associated with a dietary potassium intake of <34.6 mmol per day among 9805 participants in the first National Health and Nutrition Examination Survey (NHANES I) Epidemiological Follow-up study

Model	Hazard ratio (95% CI)	p Value
Age, energy adjusted	1.37 (1.20, 1.54)	< 0.0001
Age, race, sex and energy adjusted	1.26 (1.11, 1.45)	0.0007
Multivariate*	1.28 (1.11, 1.47)	0.0001

*Adjusted for systolic blood pressure, serum cholesterol, body mass index (BMI), history of diabetes, physical activity, education level, regular alcohol consumption, current cigarette smoking, vitamin supplement use, saturated fat intake, cholesterol intake, sodium intake, calcium intake, dietary fiber, and vitamins C and A intakes.

mental,[78,79] observational[80,81] and controlled clinical studies[82,82] in humans have investigated the association between increased calcium intake and lower blood pressure.

Animal experiments

In experimental models, a lower serum calcium level is a characteristic of the hypertensive animal.[79,84–86] In the spontaneously hypertensive rat (SHR), abnormalities in calcium metabolism are present and arise prior to the development of hypertension. Calcium supplementation not only lowers blood pressure in younger SHR, but it also has been shown in clinical trials to correct 'fixed' hypertension in older SHR. The blood-pressure-lowering effect of calcium supplementation is not limited to the SHR, having been consistently observed in a wide range of rat models.[78,87,88] Several mechanisms of action have been investigated in these models, including alterations of the sympathetic nervous system,[89,90] the renin–angiotensin system and calcium-regulating hormones,[85] calcitonin gene-related peptide, and cellular and systemic electrolyte metabolism.[91]

Observational evidence

Data from NHANES are considered an excellent source for analysis of the association between dietary intake of calcium and blood pressure because they reflect experience in a large representative sample of the US population.[92] However, results from the analysis of calcium intake on blood pressure using these data have been highly controversial; several analyses have been published with different authors coming to divergent conclusions.[93] Using data from the first NHANES study, Harlan et al.[94] concluded that dietary calcium was inversely and significantly related to diastolic blood pressure among females, but found a positive relationship in men. A significant graded association was present between lower levels of calcium intake and higher levels of blood pressure in persons without a previous diagnosis of hypertension. However, an association was not reported after adjustment for potential confounders such as age, race and sex. Using data from NHANES II, McCarron et al.[95] reported that a higher calcium intake was associated with a lower level of blood pressure levels. This analysis did not account for the complex sampling methodology used in NHANES to obtain accurate variance estimates. In a subsequent analysis of NHANES I and II by Sempos et al.,[80] which took into account the NHANES sampling methodology and adjusted for several potential confounders (including age, race, sex and BMI), no consistent relationship was identified between calcium intake and the presence of hypertension.

Evidence from cross-sectional studies is weakened by the potential for bias, including the possibility that diagnosis of hypertension leads to an alteration in dietary intake. Although most observational studies of calcium intake and blood pressure have been cross-sectional, there have been several reports from prospective cohort studies. Among 58,000 females followed from 1980 to 1984 in the Nurses' Health Study, baseline dietary calcium was inversely associated with the risk of developing hypertension.[96] Compared to women consuming <400 mg per day of calcium, those consuming ≥800 mg per day had a relative risk (95% CI) of incident of hypertension of 0.78 (0.69, 0.88). However, no association was noted between calcium intake and the incidence of hypertension within the same cohort between 1984 and 1988.[66] After 7 years of follow-up of the Western Electric Study, an inverse relationship was noted in men between dietary calcium intake and diastolic, but not systolic, blood pressure.[97] However, no association was reported after 8 years of follow-up.[98] The results from the Western Electric Study were only reported in abstract form, limiting the opportunity for additional interpretation.

A meta-analysis of observational studies by Cappuccio et al.,[99] and revised by Birkett,[100] found dietary calcium intake to be associated with modestly lower levels of systolic and diastolic blood pressures. The meta-analysis included 23 studies, of which 19 were cross-sectional, two were prospective and two were of mixed design. In this analysis, a 100 mg higher level of calcium intake per day was associated with 0.34 (95% CI: 0.46, 0.22) and 0.22 (0.32, 0.13) lower levels of systolic and diastolic blood pressure among men, and 0.15 (0.19, 0.11) and 0.05 (0.09, 0.01) among women.

Clinical trials of calcium supplementation

Dozens of clinical trials and several meta-analyses of these trials have been performed to assess whether calcium supplementation lowers blood pressure. The initial randomized controlled trials of calcium supplementation varied in size, duration, calcium supplementation and baseline calcium intake within the population. Therefore, results from meta-analyses of these trials provide more robust evidence regarding a potential association between calcium intake and blood pressure.

In 1989, Cappucio et al.[101] pooled 15 randomized clinical trials of almost 400 participants and reported no decrease in supine blood pressure among those receiving calcium supplementation (Fig. 4.4). A subsequent meta-analysis performed by Cutler and Brittain[102] found a 1.8 (0.6, 3.0) and 0.7 mmHg (−0.2, 1.5) reduction in systolic and diastolic blood pressures, respectively. A more recent meta-analysis used data from 33 randomized controlled clinical trials of calcium supplementation. In this meta-analysis, the pooled reduction (95% CI) in systolic and diastolic blood pressures for those receiving calcium supplementation was 1.27 (2.25, 0.29) and 0.24 mmHg (0.92, +0.44) greater than for those receiving placebo.[103] A small

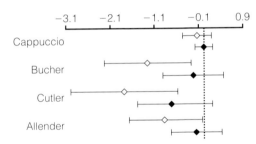

Figure 4.4

The effect of calcium supplementation on systolic ├──◇──┤ and diastolic ├──◆──┤ blood pressure from four meta-analyses. From Cappuccio *et al.*,[101] Bucher *et al.*[103] Cutler and Brittain,[102] and Allender *et al.*[82]

reduction in systolic, but not in diastolic blood pressure was also noted in a meta-analysis performed by Allender *et al.*[82] (*Fig. 4.4*).

Calcium intake and CVD outcomes

Several large cohort analyses have been conducted to investigate the association between calcium intake and risk of CVD, CHD and stroke. During 28 years of follow-up the adjusted relative risk of CVD and CHD mortality comparing the lowest to highest quintiles of calcium intake among 2605 Dutch civil servants was 1.3 (0.8, 1.9) and 0.9 (0.6, 1.6) for men, and 1.1 (0.6, 2.0) and 1.1 (0.5, 2.5) for women.[104] Additionally, among post-menopausal women in Iowa's Women's Health Study Cohort, participants who were not taking calcium supplementation, the relative risk (95% CI) of ischemic heart disease mortality was 0.63 (0.40, 0.98) for women in the highest versus lowest quintile of dietary calcium intake.[105] However, in this study, no association was found between total calcium intake and ischemic heart disease mortality. Also, calcium supplementation did not significantly lower the risk of ischemic heart disease for women with an otherwise low level of dietary calcium intake (relative risk = 0.66; 95% CI: 0.36, 1.23).

Limited evidence indicates that a higher calcium intake does not influence stroke risk among men. During the initial 8 years of the Health Professionals Follow-up study, men in the highest quintile of calcium intake had a 0.88 (0.63, 1.23) risk of stroke compared to their counterparts in the lowest quintile. Additionally, there was no association between calcium intake and stroke among 859 men and women followed for 12 years; after adjustment for age and sex, for each 10 mmol higher calcium intake the risk of stroke mortality was 0.89 (95% CI: 0.44, 1.80). However, in a subsequent study, among 85,764 women in the Nurses' Health Study, the risk of ischemic and intraparenchymal stroke was 0.72 (0.53, 0.98) and 0.56 (0.24, 1.30), respectively, for those in the highest calcium intake group compared to their counterparts in the lowest quintile.[71] In contrast, a higher quintile of calcium intake was associated with an increased risk of subarachnoid hemorrhage and was not associated with all strokes.

In summary, the overall consensus is that if calcium supplementation reduces blood pressure, its effect is minimal. The current JNC VI guidelines state that evidence does not affirm the claim that supplementation of calcium is an adequate measure to lower blood pressure. They do, however, recommend maintaining adequate calcium intake for other health purposes.

Combined dietary approaches

In addition to reduced sodium and increased potassium, other dietary factors may influence blood pressure.[106,107] In trials of vegetarian diets, replacing animal products with fruits and vegetables has reduced blood pressure among both normotensives and hypertensives.[108,109] Aspects of vegetarian diets believed to reduce blood pressure include high levels of nutrients and fiber and reduced fat.[110] However, as previously discussed, trials that have tested the ability of individual nutrients to lower blood pressure have often produced reductions in blood pressure that have been small and inconsistent. The presence of a synergistic effect such that consumption of increased amounts of these nutrients in sum results in a more substantial and important reduction in blood pressure has been proposed.[111] Also proposed is the possibility that the method of nutrient administration has an effect on blood pressure reduction. Specifically, it has been suggested that dietary supplementation may reduce blood pressure more than corresponding supplementation from food.[112] Two large rigorously conducted clinical trials have tested the effect of overall dietary patterns on blood pressure.[13,111]

Dietary Approaches to Stop Hypertension (DASH)[111]

The Dietary Approaches to Stop Hypertension (DASH) clinical trial randomized 459 adults with systolic blood pressures <160 mmHg and diastolic blood pressures between 80 and 95 mmHg to receive one of three diets: (a) a control diet that was considered to be low in fruits and vegetables with a fat content typical of the American diet; (b) a diet rich in fruit and vegetables but retaining the same fat intake as the control diet; or (c) a 'combined' diet rich in fruits and vegetables with reduced saturated and total fat. In the control diet and the diet rich in fruits and vegetables, 16, 13 and 8% of caloric intake was derived from saturated, monounsaturated and polyunsaturated fats, respectively. Additionally, 48 and 15% of caloric intake were derived form carbohydrates and protein, respectively. In contrast, caloric intake for the combined diet included 6% from saturated fats, 13% from monounsaturated fats, 8% from polyunsaturated fats, 55% from carbohydrates and 18% from protein. The macronutrient and mineral composition of the three diets are shown in *Table 4.3*. Within each of the three

Table 4.3 Dietary composition of the control, fruits and vegetables, and combination diets in the Dietary Approaches to Stop Hypertension (DASH) clinical trial

Nutrients	Control diet		Fruit and vegetables diet		DASH combination diet	
	Target	Actual*	Target	Actual*	Target	Actual*
Cholesterol (mg per day)	300	233	300	184	150	151
Fiber (g per day)	9	NA†	31	NA†	31	NA†
Potassium (mg per day)	1700	1752	4700	4101	4700	4415
Magnesium (mg per day)	165	176	500	423	500	480
Calcium (mg per day)	450	443	450	534	1240	1265
Sodium (mg per day)	3000	3028	3000	2816	3000	2859
Food group (servings per day)						
Fruits and juices	1.6		5.2		5.2	
Vegetables	2.0		3.3		4.4	
Grains	8.2		6.9		7.5	
Low-fat dairy	0.1		0.0		2.0	
Regular-fat dairy	0.4		0.3		0.7	
Nuts, seeds, legumes	0.0		0.6		0.7	
Beef, pork, ham	1.5		1.8		0.5	
Poultry	0.8		0.4		0.6	
Fish	0.2		0.3		0.6	
Fats, oils	5.8		5.3		2.5	
Snacks/sweets	4.1		1.4		0.7	

*Values are based on chemical analyses of the menus prepared during the validation phase and during the trial; † not applicable.
Modified from Appel et al.[111]

study arms, three meals a day and in-between meal snacks were provided to each study participant. Sodium intake and body weight were maintained at constant levels during follow-up.

The systolic and diastolic blood pressure among those receiving the diet high in fruits and vegetables declined by 2.8 (4.7, 0.9) and 1.1 mmHg (2.4, 0.3), respectively, more than those on the control diet. The relative reduction in systolic and diastolic blood pressure was 5.5 (7.4, 3.7) and 3.0 mmHg (4.3, 1.6) greater for those receiving the combination diet compared to their counterparts receiving the control diet. The effect of these diets was larger in magnitude among persons with hypertension. Compared to hypertensives in the control group, hypertensives receiving the fruits and vegetables and combination diet had a 7.2 (11.4, 3.0) and 11.4 mmHg (15.9, 6.9) larger reduction in systolic blood pressure and 2.8 (4.7, 0.9) and 5.5 mmHg (8.2, 2.7) larger reductions in diastolic blood pressure. Additionally, blood pressure reductions were seen within 2 weeks of initiating the diet and continued through to the completion of the study. The DASH combination diet provided reductions in blood pressure similar to those seen in clinical trials of drug monotherapy among persons with mild hypertension. It is worth noting that the blood pressure reductions in this randomized controlled trial occurred in the setting of stable weight, a steady level of sodium intake (3 g per day), and consumption of two or fewer alcoholic beverages per day. The DASH combination diet may provide a method to prevent the need for drug therapy among persons with mild hypertension.

Reduced sodium and the DASH combined diet[13]

Subsequent to the initial DASH trial, the combination diet was recommended in national guidelines. However, the DASH clinical trial did not investigate the benefit of sodium reduction. Therefore, the DASH collaborative study group conducted a second controlled trial. This randomized controlled trial had two primary aims. First, to determine whether reduction in dietary sodium intake to levels below the currently recommended level of 100 mmol per day lowers blood pressure more than lowering sodium intake to the current recommended guidelines was tested. The second goal was to assess whether the DASH combined diet has the ability to lower blood pressure in the context of a low sodium intake. Eligibility criteria were similar to that for the first DASH study; with regards to blood pressure, inclusion in the trial was limited to those with systolic and diastolic blood pressures of 120–159 and 80–95 mmHg, respectively. Details of the study design have been published.[113] In brief, the study design of DASH sodium dictated that each participant was randomized to either the DASH or control diet and subsequently spent 30 days receiving each of the three sodium level diets in a crossover fashion.

Compared to the control diet, the DASH diet resulted in significantly

Table 4.4 The effect of sodium reduction on systolic and diastolic blood pressures presented separately for clinical trial participants receiving the control and combined DASH diet

Sodium reduction	Control diet		Combined DASH diet	
	High sodium to medium sodium	Medium sodium to low sodium	High sodium to medium sodium	Medium sodium to low sodium
Systolic blood pressure (mmHg)	−2.1 (−3.4, −0.8)	−4.6 (−5.9, −3.2)	−1.3 (−2.6, 0.0)	−1.7 (−3.0, −0.4)
Diastolic blood pressure (mmHg)	−1.1 (−1.9, −0.2)	−2.4 (−3.3, −1.5)	−0.6 (−1.5, 0.2)	−1.0 (−1.9, −0.1)

Table 4.5   Differences in the change in systolic and diastolic blood pressures within the three sodium levels between persons randomized to the combined DASH versus control diet

	High sodium	Medium sodium	Low sodium
Systolic blood pressure (mmHg)	−5.9 (−8.0, −3.7)	−5.0 (−7.6, −2.5)	−2.2 (−4.4, −0.1)
Diastolic blood pressure (mmHg)	−2.9 (−4.3, −1.5)	−2.5 (−0.8, −4.1)	−1.0 (−2.5, 0.4)

lower systolic blood pressure at every sodium level (*Table 4.4*). Additionally, the DASH diet significantly lowered diastolic blood pressure for those in the high and medium sodium categories, and a non-significant reduction in the low sodium category (*Table 4.5*). There was a graded response with greater reductions in sodium intake producing lower systolic and diastolic blood pressures, within both the control and DASH diets. The effect of dietary sodium reduction was approximately twice as great in the control compared to the DASH diet. The results of this trial provide strong evidence that a diet high in fruits and vegetables can lower blood pressure regardless of sodium intake. Equally important, however, is the observation that a reduction in sodium intake resulted in a lowering of blood pressure among persons eating either the typical American diet or a healthy diet that was high in fruits and vegetables. Finally, a synergistic blood pressure lowering effect was noted such that persons consuming both a diet low in sodium and high in fruits and vegetables had sharper reductions than either single approach alone.

Conclusions

JNC VI guidelines recommend dietary modification as a valuable means to treat and prevent hypertension. Even when dietary modification is not a singular cure, there is evidence that this approach can reduce the quantity of antihypertensive medication needed. Overall, the balance of evidence supports the JNC VI recommendations. Specifically, consistent evidence from clinical trials supports the efficacy of sodium reduction and potassium supplementation in lowering blood pressure. Although, calcium supplementation may not be effective in lowering blood pressure, it does provide other health benefits and an adequate intake should be provided. Finally, recent evidence from the two DASH controlled trials provides evidence that an overall dietary approach, including high nutrient intake along with low sodium intake, has the ability to lower blood pressure as much as drug monotherapy.

References

1. Cappuccio FP, MacGregor GA. Non-pharmacological treatment of hypertension (letter; comment). Lancet 1994; 344: 884.

2. Beilin LJ. Key issues regarding lifestyle in the prevention and treatment of hypertension. Clin Exp Hypertens 1996; 18: 473–487.

3. Joint National Committee (JNC). The sixth report of the Joint National Committee. Nat Inst Health 1997; 1–70.

4. He J, Bazzano LA. Effects of lifestyle modification on treatment and prevention of hypertension. Curr Opin Nephrol Hypertens 2000; 9: 267–271.

5. Ambard L, Beaujard E. Causes de l'hypertension artérielle. Arch Gen Med 1904; 1: 520–533.

6. Kempner W. Treatment of kidney disease and hypertensive vascular disease with rice diet. Am J Med 1948; 4: 545–577.

7. Dahl LK. Possible role of salt intake in the development of essential hypertension. In: Bock KD, Cottier PT, eds. Essential hypertension. Berlin, Germany: Springer-Verlag, 1960, 53–65.

8. Swales JD. Dietary salt and hypertension. Lancet 1980; 1: 1177–1179.

9. MacGregor GA. Sodium and potassium intake and high blood pressure. Eur Heart J 1987; 8 (suppl B): 3–8.

10. Weinberger MH. Sodium chloride and blood pressure (editorial). N Engl J Med 1987; 317: 1084–1086.

11. Denton D, Weisinger R, Munday NI et al. The effect of increased salt intake on blood pressure of chimpanzees (see comments). Nat Med 1995; 1: 1009–1016.

12. Stamler R, Shipley M, Elliott P et al. Higher blood pressure in adults with less education. Some explanations from INTERSALT. Hypertension 1992; 19: 237–241.

13. Sacks FM, Svetkey LP, Vollmer WM et al. Effects on blood pressure of reduced dietary sodium and the Dietary Approaches to Stop Hypertension (DASH) diet. N Engl J Med 2001; 344: 3–10.

14. Law MR, Frost CD, Wald NJ. By how much does dietary salt reduction lower blood pressure? III – Analysis of data from trials of salt reduction (published erratum appears in BMJ 1991; 302: 939). BMJ 1991; 302: 819–824.

15. Moore TJ, Malarick C, Olmedo A, Klein RC. Salt restriction lowers resting blood pressure but not 24-h ambulatory blood pressure (see comments). Am J Hypertens 1991; 4: 410–415.

16. Cutler JA, Follmann D, Allender PS. Randomized trials of sodium reduction: an overview. Am J Clin Nutr 1997; 65: 643S–651S.

17. Whelton PK, Kumanyika SK, Cook NR et al. Efficacy of non-pharmacologic interventions in adults with high-normal blood pressure: results from phase 1 of the Trials of Hypertension Prevention. Trials of Hypertension Prevention Collaborative Research Group. Am J Clin Nutr 1997; 65: 652S–660S.

18. He J, Whelton PK. Role of sodium reduction in the treatment and prevention of hypertension. Curr Opin Cardiol 1997; 12: 202–207.

19. Liu K, Cooper R, McKeever J et al. Assessment of the association between habitual salt intake and high blood pressure: methodological problems. Am J Epidemiol 1979; 110: 219–226.

20. Elliott P, Marmot M. International

studies of salt and blood pressure. Ann Clin Res 1984; 16 (suppl 43): 67–71.

21. Elliott P. Observational studies of salt and blood pressure. Hypertension 1991; 17: I3–I8.

22. Weinberger MH. Salt sensitivity as a predictor of hypertension. Am J Hypertens 1991; 4: 615S–616S.

23. Schachter J, Harper PH, Radin ME et al. Comparison of sodium and potassium intake with excretion. Hypertension 1980; 2: 695–699.

24. Svetkey LP, McKeown SP, Wilson AF. Heritability of salt sensitivity in black Americans. Hypertension 1996; 28: 854–858.

25. He J, Whelton PK. Epidemiology and prevention of hypertension. Med Clin North Am 1997; 81: 1077–1097.

26. Massry SG, Coburn JW. The hormonal and non-hormonal control of renal excretion of calcium and magnesium. Nephron 1973; 10: 66–112.

27. Pietinen PI, Findley TW, Clausen JD et al. Studies in community nutrition: estimation of sodium output. Prev Med 1976; 5: 400–407.

28. Liu K, Dyer AR, Cooper RS et al. Can overnight urine replace 24-hour urine collection to assess salt intake? Hypertension 1979; 1: 529–536.

29. Liu K, Cooper R, Soltero I, Stamler J. Variability in 24-hour urine sodium excretion in children. Hypertension 1979; 1: 631–636.

30. Gleibermann L. Blood pressure and dietary salt in human populations. Ecol Food Nutr 1973; 2: 143–156.

31. Froment A, Milon H, Gravier C. [Relationship of sodium intake and arterial hypertension. Contribution of geographical epidemi-ology (author's translation)]. Rev Épidémiol Santé Publique 1979; 27: 437–454.

32. Simpson FO. Blood pressure and sodium intake. In: Anon, ed. Handbook of hypertension, Volume 6: Epidemiology of hypertension. Amsterdam: Elsevier, 1985, 175–190.

33. Elliott P, Marmot M, Dyer A et al. The INTERSALT study: main results, conclusions and some implications. Clin Exp Hypertens [A] 1989; 11: 1025–1034.

34. Morgenstein H. Uses of ecologic analysis in epidemiologic research. Am J Pub Health 1982; 72: 1336–1344.

35. Piantadosi S, Byar D, Green S. The ecological fallacy. Am J Epidemiol 1988; 127: 893–904.

36. Greenland S. Divergent biases in ecological and individual-level studies. Stats Med 1992; 11: 1209–1223.

37. Elliott P, Stamler J, Nichols R et al. INTERSALT revisited: further analyses of 24 hour sodium excretion and blood pressure within and across populations. INTERSALT Cooperative Research Group (see comments; published erratum appears in BMJ 1997; 315: 458). BMJ 1996; 312: 1249–1253.

38. Parfrey PS, Vandenburg MJ, Wright P et al. Blood pressure and hormonal changes following alteration in dietary sodium and potassium in mild essential hypertension. Lancet 1981; 1: 59–63.

39. Staessen JA, Lijnen P, Thijs L, Fagard R. Salt and blood pressure in community-based intervention trials. Am J Clin Nutr 1997; 65: 661S–670S.

40. Cappuccio FP, Markandu ND, Carney C et al. Double-blind randomised trial of modest salt restriction in older people (see

comments). Lancet 1997; 350: 850–854.

41. Midgley JP, Matthew AG, Greenwood CM, Logan AG. Effect of reduced dietary sodium on blood pressure: a meta-analysis of randomized controlled trials. JAMA 1996; 275: 1590–1597.

42. He J, Ogden LG, Vupputuri S et al. Dietary sodium intake and subsequent risk of cardiovascular disease in overweight adults (see comments). JAMA 1999; 282: 2027–2034.

43. Alderman MH, Madhaven S, Cohen H et al. Low urinary sodium is associated with greater risk of myocardial infarction among treated hypertensive men (see comments). Hypertension 1995; 25: 1144–1152.

44. Stamler J, Rose G, Stamler R et al. INTERSALT study findings. Public health and medical care implications. Hypertension 1989; 14: 570–577.

45. Addison WL. The use of sodium chloride, potassium chloride, sodium bromide, and potassium bromide in cases of arterial hypertension which are amenable to potassium chloride. Can Med Assoc J 1928; 18: 281–285.

46. Tannen RL. Effects of potassium on blood pressure control. Ann Intern Med 1983; 98: 773–780.

47. Tannen RL. The influence of potassium on blood pressure. Kidney Int 1987; 22 (suppl): S242–S248.

48. West ML, Sonnenberg H, Veress A, Halperin ML. The relationship between the plasma potassium concentration and renal potassium excretion in the adrenalectomized rat. Clin Sci 1987; 72: 577–583.

49. He J, Whelton PK. What is the role of dietary sodium and potassium in hypertension and target organ injury? Am J Med Sci 1999; 317: 152–159.

50. Whelton PK, Buring J, Borhani NO et al. The effect of potassium supplementation in persons with a high-normal blood pressure. Results from phase I of the Trials of Hypertension Prevention (TOHP). Trials of Hypertension Prevention (TOHP) Collaborative Research Group. Ann Epidemiol 1995; 5: 85–95.

51. Freed SC. Hypotension in the rat following limitation of potassium intake. Science 1950; 112: 788–789.

52. Paller MS, Linas SL. Role of vasopressin in support of blood pressure in potassium deficient rats. Kidney Int 1983; 24: 342–347.

53. Bahler RC, Rakita L. Cardiovascular function in potassium-depleted dogs. Am Heart J 1971; 81: 650–657.

54. Reid WD, Laragh JH. Sodium and potassium intake, blood pressure and pressor response to angiotensin. Proc Soc Exp Biol Med 1965; 120: 26–29.

55. Campbell WB, Schmitz JM. Effect of alterations in dietary potassium on the pressor and steroidogenic effects of angiotensins II and III. Endocrinology 1978; 103: 2098–2104.

56. Kaplan NM. Calcium and potassium in the treatment of essential hypertension. Semin Nephrol 1988; 8: 176–184.

57. Kaplan NM, Ram CV. Potassium supplements for hypertension (editorial; comment). N Engl J Med 1990; 322: 623–624.

58. Anon. INTERSALT Study: an international co-operative study on the relation of blood pressure to electrolyte excretion in populations. I. Design and methods.

The INTERSALT Co-operative Research Group. J Hypertens 1986; 4: 781–787.

59. Krishna GG. Effect of potassium intake on blood pressure. J Am Soc Nephrol 1990; 1: 43–52.

60. Linas SL. The role of potassium in the pathogenesis and treatment of hypertension (clinical conference). Kidney Int 1991; 39: 771–786.

61. Langford HG. Potassium in hypertension. Postgrad Med 1983; 73: 227–233.

62. Langford HG. Dietary potassium and hypertension: epidemiologic data. Ann Intern Med 1983; 98: 770–772.

63. Krishna GG. Role of potassium in the pathogenesis of hypertension. Am J Med Sci 1994; 307 (suppl 1): S21–S25.

64 Watson RL, Langford HG. Weight, urinary electrolytes and blood pressure – results of several community based studies. J Chronic Dis 1982; 32: 909–918.

65. Sacks FM, Willett WC, Smith A et al. Effect on blood pressure of potassium, calcium, and magnesium in women with low habitual intake. Hypertension 1998; 31: 131–138.

66. Ascherio A, Rimm EB, Giovannucci EL et al. A prospective study of nutritional factors and hypertension among US men. Circulation 1992; 86: 1475–1484.

67. Whelton PK, He J, Cutler JA et al. Effects of oral potassium on blood pressure. Meta-analysis of randomized controlled clinical trials (see comments). JAMA 1997; 277: 1624–1632.

68. Cappuccio FP, MacGregor GA. Does potassium supplementation lower blood pressure? A meta-analysis of published trials. J Hypertens 1991; 9: 465–473.

69. Xie JX, Sasaki S, Joossens JV. The relationship between urinary cations obtained from the INTERSALT study and cerebrovascular mortality. J Hum Hypertens 1992; 6: 17–21.

70. Yamori Y, Nara Y, Mizushima S. Nutritional factors for stroke and major cardiovascular diseases: international epidemiological comparison of dietary prevention. Health Rep 1994; 6: 22–27.

71. Iso H, Stampfer MJ, Manson JE et al. Prospective study of calcium, potassium, and magnesium intake and risk of stroke in women. Stroke 1999; 30: 1772–1779.

72. Ascherio A, Rimm EB, Hernan MA et al. Intake of potassium, magnesium, calcium, and fiber and risk of stroke among US men. Circulation 1998; 98: 1198–1204.

73. Khaw KT, Barrett-Connor E. Dietary potassium and stroke-associated mortality. A 12-year prospective population study. N Engl J Med 1987; 316: 235–240.

74. Bazzano LA, He J, Ogden LG et al. Dietary potassium intake and risk of stroke in US men and women: NHANES I epidemiologic follow-up study. Stroke 2001; 32: 1473–1480

75. Stitt FW, Clayton DG, Crawford MD, Morris JN. Clinical and biochemical indicators of cardiovascular disease among men living in hard and soft water areas. Lancet 1973; 1: 122–126.

76. Neri LC, Johansen HL. Water hardness and cardiovascular mortality. Ann N Y Acad Sci 1978; 304: 203–221.

77. Schroeder HA. Relationship between mortality from cardiovascular disease and treated water supplies; variation in states and 163 largest municipalities of

the United States. JAMA 1960; 172: 1902–1908.

78. Porsti I, Arvola P, Wuorela H, Vapaatalo H. High calcium diet augments vascular potassium relaxation in hypertensive rats. Hypertension 1992; 19: 85–92.

79. Porsti I, Makynen H. Dietary calcium intake: effects on central blood pressure control. Semin Nephrol 1995; 15: 550–563.

80. Sempos C, Cooper R, Kovar MG et al. Dietary calcium and blood pressure in National Health and Nutrition Examination Surveys I and II. Hypertension 1986; 8: 1067–1074.

81. McCarron DA, Morris CD. Epidemiological evidence associating dietary calcium and calcium metabolism with blood pressure. Am J Nephrol 1986; 6 (suppl 1): 3–9.

82. Allender PS, Cutler JA, Follman D et al. Dietary calcium and blood pressure: a meta-analysis of randomized clinical trials (see comments). Ann Intern Med 1996; 124: 825–831.

83. Cappuccio FP, Markandu ND, Singer DR et al. Does oral calcium supplementation lower high blood pressure? A double blind study. J Hypertens 1987; 5: 67–71.

84. Itokawa Y, Tanaka C, Fujiwara M. Changes in body temperature and blood pressure in rats with calcium and magnesium deficiencies. J Appl Physiol 1974; 37: 835–839.

85. Hatton DC, McCarron DA. Dietary calcium and blood pressure in experimental models of hypertension. A review. Hypertension 1994; 23: 513–530.

86. Hatton DC, Scrogin KE, Metz JA, McCarron DA. Dietary calcium alters blood pressure reactivity in spontaneously hypertensive rats. Hypertension 1989; 13: 622–629.

87. Peuler JD, Morgan DA, Mark AL. High calcium diet reduces blood pressure in Dahl salt-sensitive rats by neural mechanisms. Hypertension 1987; 9 (suppl III): III159–III165.

88. Peuler JD, Schelper RL. Partial protection from salt-induced stroke and mortality by high oral calcium in hypertensive rats. Stroke 1992; 23: 532–538.

89. Reid JL. Hypertension and the brain. BMJ 1994; 50: 371–380.

90. Oparil S, Wyss JM, Yang RH. Dietary Ca^{2+} prevents NaCl-sensitive hypertension in spontaneously hypertensive rats by a sympatholytic mechanism. Am J Hypertens 1990; 3: 179S–188S.

91. Drueke TB. Mechanisms of action of calcium absorption: factors that influence bioavailability. In: Langford HG, Levine B, Ellenbogen L, eds. Nutrition factors in hypertension. Alan R Liss: New York, 1990, 155–173.

92. Harlan WR, Harlan LC. An epidemiological perspective on dietary electrolytes and hypertension. J Hypertens 1986; 4 (suppl 4): S334–S339.

93. Morris C, McCarron DA. Dietary calcium intake in hypertension. Hypertension 1987; 10: 350–353.

94. Harlan WR, Hull AL, Schmouder RL et al. Blood pressure and nutrition in adults. The National Health and Nutrition Examination Survey. Am J Epidemiol 1984; 120: 17–28.

95. McCarron DA, Morris CD, Henry HJ, Stanton JL. Blood pressure and nutrient intake in the United States. Science 1984; 224: 1392–1398.

96. Witteman JC, Willett WC, Stampfer MJ et al. A prospective study of nutritional factors and

hypertension among US women. Circulation 1989; 80: 1320–1327.

97. Zhang HY, Liu K, Shekelle R. The impact of calcium intake on incidence of elevated blood pressure: the Western Electric Study (abstract). Am J Epidemiol 1988; 128: 916–917.

98. Nichaman M, Shekelle R, Paul O. Diet, alcohol, and blood pressure in the Western Electric Study (abstract). Am J Epidemiol 1984; 120: 469–470.

99. Cappuccio FP, Elliott P, Allender PS et al. Epidemiologic association between dietary calcium intake and blood pressure: a meta-analysis of published data. Am J Epidemiol 1995; 142: 935–945.

100. Birkett NJ. Comments on a meta-analysis of the relation between dietary calcium intake and blood pressure. Am J Epidemiol 1998; 148: 223–228.

101. Cappuccio FP, Siani A, Strazzullo P. Oral calcium supplementation and blood pressure: an overview of randomized controlled trials. J Hypertens 1989; 7: 941–946.

102. Cutler JA, Brittain E. Calcium and blood pressure. An epidemiologic perspective. Am J Hypertens 1990; 3: 137S–146S.

103. Bucher HC, Cook RJ, Guyatt GH et al. Effects of dietary calcium supplementation on blood pressure. A meta-analysis of randomized controlled trials (see comments). JAMA 1996; 275: 1016–1022.

104. Van der Vijver LP, van der Waal MA, Weterings KG et al. Calcium intake and 28-year cardiovascular and coronary heart disease mortality in Dutch civil servants. Int J Epidemiol 1992; 21: 36–39.

105. Bostick RM, Kushi LH, Wu Y et al. Relation of calcium, vitamin D, and dairy food intake to ischemic heart disease mortality among postmenopausal women. Am J Epidemiol 1999; 149: 151–161.

106. Stamler J, Caggiula A, Grandits GA et al. Relationship to blood pressure of combinations of dietary macronutrients. Findings of the Multiple Risk Factor Intervention Trial (MRFIT). Circulation 1996; 94: 2417–2423.

107. Obarzanek E, Velletri PA, Cutler JA. Dietary protein and blood pressure. JAMA 1996; 275: 1598–1603.

108. Sacks FM, Rosner B, Kass EH. Blood pressure in vegetarians. Am J Epidemiol 1974; 100: 390–398.

109. Rouse IL, Beilin LJ, Armstrong BK, Vandongen R. Blood-pressure-lowering effect of a vegetarian diet: controlled trial in normotensive subjects. Lancet 1983; 1: 5–10.

110. Margetts BM, Beilin LJ, Vandongen R, Armstrong BK. Vegetarian diet in mild hypertension: a randomised controlled trial. BMJ (Clin Res Ed) 1986; 293: 1468–1471.

111. Appel LJ, Moore TJ, Obarzanek E et al. A clinical trial of the effects of dietary patterns on blood pressure. DASH Collaborative Research Group (see comments). N Engl J Med 1997; 336: 1117–1124.

112. Willett W, Buzzard M. Foods and nutrients. In: Willett WC, ed. Nutritional epidemiology. Oxford University Press: Oxford, 1998, 18–32.

113. Svetkey LP, Sacks FM, Obarzanek E et al. The DASH Diet, Sodium Intake and Blood Pressure Trial (DASH-sodium): rationale and design. DASH-Sodium Collaborative Research Group. J Am Diet Assoc 1999; 99 (suppl): S96–S104.

5
Management of proteinuric nephropathies

Michael Schömig and Eberhard Ritz

Mechanisms of hypertension in renal disease

Transplantation experiments show that hypertension goes with the kidney, i.e. when kidneys of genetically hypertension prone rats (SHRsp) are transplanted into normotensive compatible recipients (i.e. recipients which are unable to launch a rejection crisis), blood pressure increases continuously with time.[1] This is remarkable, since apparently a transplanted kidney which is genetically programmed for hypertension is able to override blood pressure regulation in a recipient, the circulatory regulation of which is programmed to maintain normotension. This phenomenon is not unique to the rat but has also been observed in humans.[2] Several patients who had become dialysis dependent because of hypertensive renal damage in the absence of primary renal disease had received the kidneys of normotensive donors. This often resulted in normotension despite no antihypertensive treatment.

Against this background it is not surprising that hypertension is common in the patient whose kidneys are diseased. Several mechanisms are operative and explain the maintenance of hypertension in chronic renal disease. Firstly, it has been known for decades that blood pressure in the renal patient is salt sensitive. Guyton[3] proposed that salt retention in these patients is due to a shift in the blood pressure/natriuresis relationship: he hypothesized that salt and water intake results in expansion of the plasma and extracellular volumes, thus acutely increasing cardiac output and blood pressure. In the long run, however, the need to keep tissue perfusion constant should cause vasoconstriction by some unknown mechanism, thus raising peripheral resistance. There is also evidence that in renal patients salt loading causes a more pronounced increase in arterial pressure than in controls.[4] Salt dependence of blood pressure in renal patients provides a rationale for dietary sodium restriction and the use of diuretic agents in the treatment of hypertensive renal patients.

A second factor is inappropriate activity of the renin–angiotensin system. This system is activated early on, even in normotensive young patients with hereditary renal disease renin is increased.[5] One of the mechanisms increasing the activity of the renin system is patchy non-homogenous ischemia resulting from damage to some preglomerular vessels in the kidney. Such ischemia will drive renin secretion, but despite the elevation of systemic blood pressure stenosed preglomerular vessels interfere with feedback inhibition of renin secretion. As a result, plasma renin activity is inappropriately high.[6] This is not the only mechanism stimulating renin secretion. For instance, in the diseased kidney, local production of angiotensin II is seen outside of the juxtaglomerular apparatus. This may explain the paradox that angiotensin-converting-enzyme (ACE) inhibitors attenuate renal damage, even in individuals with a suppressed circulating renin system.[7]

Thirdly, although it had been known for some time that sympathicoplegic agents, e.g. clonidine, are uniquely effective in the renal patient, clear evidence for sympathetic overactivity in uremic patients has been provided only recently.[8] Sympathetic overactivity disappeared after bilateral nephrectomy, suggesting that the diseased kidney is the cause of sympathetic activation. This hypothesis has been directly documented in renal damage models, i.e. subtotal nephrectomy[9] or phenol application to the kidney. As shown in *Fig. 5.1*, in subtotally nephrectomized rats interruption of afferent nerve traffic by sectioning the dorsal roots markedly attenuated the increase in blood pressure. Sympathetic overactivity may also be a novel therapeutic target to attenuate progression of renal failure: in subtotally nephrectomized rats low doses of sympathicoplegic agents that failed to lower blood pressure by telemetric blood pressure measurements inhibited the development of glomerulosclerosis and reduced albumin excretion.[10] The same was seen in normotensive microalbuminuric type 1 diabetic patients.[11]

There are a number of other potential factors such as loss of renal vasodepressor factors (medullipin), inhibition of the synthesis of vasodilatatory nitric oxide or increased intracellular calcium concentrations. However, these abnormalities are currently not susceptible to intervention.

Role of blood pressure in the genesis of glomerular injury and proteinuria

The overriding importance of hypertension for progression of renal disease is illustrated by experiments of Bidani et al.,[12] according to which little or no progression is seen in renal-damage models when systemic hypertension is not present. Conversely, there is overwhelming evidence to document a beneficial effect of blood pressure lowering on progression in hypertensive individuals with renal disease.

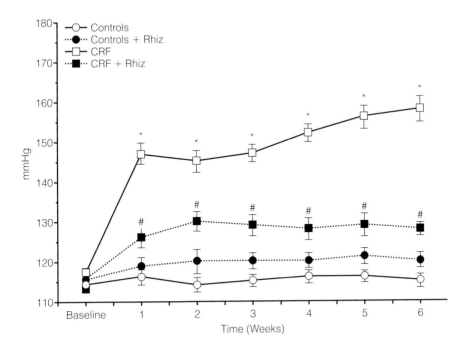

Figure 5.1

Blood pressure in subtotally nephrectomized rats with chronic renal failure (CRF) and
influence of dorsal rhizotomy (Rhiz). (After Campese and Kogosov.[9])

One feature of progression is elevation of intraglomerular pressures
secondary to afferent vasodilatation, as documented in experiments
using servonulling techniques. Such glomerular capillary hypertension
results from afferent vasodilatation and reflects greater transmission of
aortic pressure to the glomerular microcirculation. Further mechanisms
causing glomerular damage in progressive renal injury are mechanical
distension of capillaries and basal membranes, increasing pore size and
filtration of protein. Recently, the podocyte, i.e. the glomerular epithelial
cell, has been identified as a key cell in the development of glomerular
damage. It may be susceptible to mechanical damage from distension
and chemical change by reactive oxygen species or angiotensin II.[13]

In the past there has been much discussion as to whether ACE
inhibitors are superior to alternative antihypertensive agents in halting
progression. In the seminal study of Anderson et al.,[14] ACE inhibitors
were found to be superior to triple therapy comprising reserpin,
hydrochlorothiazide and hydralazin. It has been concluded that ACE
inhibitors preferentially vasodilate the efferent vessel thus reducing
glomerular pressure at any given level of systemic blood pressure. More

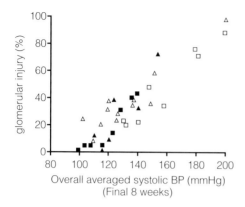

Figure 5.2

Correlation of percentage glomeruli with injury in groups of rats with subtotal nephrectomy. Systolic blood pressure (BP) was telemetrically recorded. No treatment (□), enalapril (■), triple therapy comprising reserpin, hydralazine, and hydrochlorothiazide in low doses (△), triple therapy in high doses (▲). The graph shows an excellent correlation between overall average systolic blood pressure and glomerular injury. (After Anderson *et*

recently, it has been proposed that the difference between ACE inhibitors and other agents may be related to the different effect on average circadian blood pressure,[15] as illustrated in *Fig. 5.2*, where glomerular injury is plotted as a function of time-averaged systolic blood pressure. ACE inhibitors are exactly on the regression line that describes the effects of all available antihypertensive agents. Nevertheless, there are also strong arguments for blood pressure-independent effects of ACE inhibitors. These include effects on glomerular size and structure,[16] as well as effects on proteinuria which is more effectively reduced by ACE inhibitors than by alternative antihypertensive agents.[17,18] ACE inhibitors also interfere with proliferation of glomerular cells and expression of cytokines, particularly transforming growth factor-beta (TGF-β-1).[19]

The action of calcium-channel blockers (CCB) is less consistent and more controversial. In a renal ablation[20] and the two-kidney one-clip-models,[21] aggravation of proteinuria and accelerated development of glomerulosclerosis were noted with verapamil and nitrenidipine, respectively. In these studies, systemic blood pressure was not normalized; however, it is possible that afferent vasodilatation by CCB in the presence of systemic hypertension aggravated glomerular hypertension. When blood pressure was effectively lowered, less development of glomerulosclerosis was noted in animals that were treated with CCB, e.g. after uninephrectomy,[22] DOCA salt hypertension[23] and spontaneous glomerulosclerosis in the SHRsp rat.[24]

Natural history of progression in proteinuric diabetic and non-diabetic renal disease

It had been recognized that in many, but not all, patients with renal disease glomerular filtration rate (GFR) is lost at a constant rate. Mitch *et al.*[25] showed that 1/serum creatinine increases linearly with time in most patients with renal disease.[25] Amongst the predictors of risk of progression, blood pressure and the rate of protein excretion are most prominent. Although it had been suspected decades ago that high blood pressure is related to loss of renal function, definite evidence from observational studies has only been forthcoming relatively recently in diabetic[26,27] and non-diabetic renal disease.[28,29]

Using the transplanted kidney as a model of vascular injury to the kidney, Opelz *et al.*[30] noted that blood pressure 1 year after transplantation was a powerful predictor of 8-year graft survival, as illustrated in *Fig. 5.3*. In this study systolic blood pressure was more predictive than diastolic blood pressure. It is also of note that at any given rate of average 24-hour arterial pressure individuals with reduced night-time decrease of blood pressure (non-dippers) had a more rapid loss of GFR than dippers.[31,32]

The rate of urinary protein excretion is highly predictive of renal outcome. There is strong interaction between albuminuria or proteinuria on the one hand and blood pressure on the other (*Fig. 5.4*). Mogensen[33] assessed urinary albumin excretion as a function of clinic blood pressure in type 1 diabetic patients. The average annual percentage increase in urinary albumin excretion increased steadily with higher blood pressures. It is of interest that no such increase was seen when mean arterial

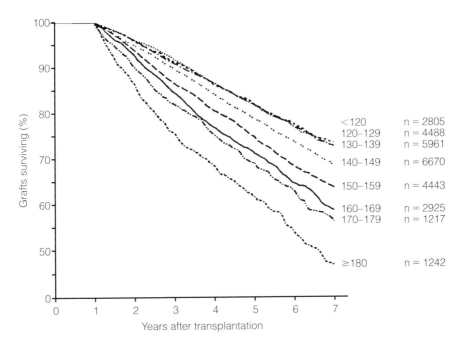

Figure 5.3

Association of systolic blood pressure at 1 year with subsequent graft survival in recipients of cadaver kidney transplants. (After Opelz *et al.*[30])

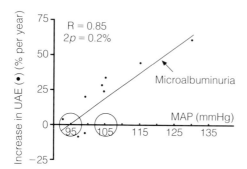

Figure 5.4

Relation between mean arterial pressure (MAP) and annual percentage increase of urinary albumin excretion (UAE) in patients with type 1 diabetes. (After Mogensen.[33])

pressure was as low as 90–95 mmHg (see below). Not only is proteinuria a predictor of progression, but in both diabetic[34] and non-diabetic[35] renal disease patients those in whom the acute antiproteinuric effect of antihypertensive agents is most marked also have the greatest attenuation of the rate of loss of GFR.

Intervention studies in diabetic and non-diabetic nephropathy

A correlation between blood pressure and rate of progression is, of course, not definite proof of causality: diseased kidneys that are intrinsically more prone to progression might coincidentally also cause a greater increase in blood pressure. To prove causality, intervention studies were necessary and these were first performed in diabetic nephropathy.[26,27] Meanwhile, several studies are also reported on non-diabetic renal disease[36,37] which document an attenuation of the rate of loss of GFR. *Figure 5.5* shows the relation between achieved blood pressure and rate of loss of GFR in proteinuric and non-proteinuric renal disease.[36] The effect is obviously most impressive in proteinuric renal disease. The marked effect of urinary protein excretion on the rate of loss of GFR and the reversal by ACE inhibitors have also been confirmed in the REIN study.[38] In non-proteinuric renal disease, particularly in autosomal dominant polycystic kidney disease (ADPKD), there is no evidence of a beneficial effect of aggressive lowering of blood pressure in advanced renal failure,[36] but studies on antihypertensive treatment in earlier stages of the disease are currently ongoing.

If albuminuria or proteinuria is accepted as a surrogate marker to monitor the effect on progression, it is of note that if one lowers blood pressure the rate of albumin or protein excretion decreases in diabetic[26,27] and non-diabetic renal disease.[29] In a meta-analysis (*Fig. 5.6*), Weidmann et al.[39] showed that, with respect to reducing proteinuria in diabetic patients, ACE inhibitors were superior to alternative antihypertensive

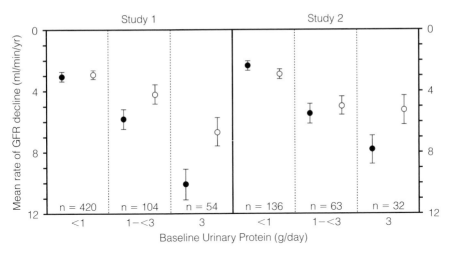

Figure 5.5

Decline in the glomerular filtration rate (GFR) according to baseline urinary protein excretion and blood pressure group in studies 1 (intake 1.3 g of protein per kilogram of body weight per day) and 2 (0.58 g of protein per kilogram of body weight per day). ●, Low blood pressure (mean arterial pressure 92 mmHg); ○, high blood pressure (mean arterial pressure 107 mmHg). (After Klahr et al.[36])

agents. It is of note, however, that ACE inhibitors were superior only when blood pressure was not lowered at all or lowered only modestly. If blood pressure was reduced by >20%, however, ACE inhibitors lost their superiority over alternative antihypertensive agents and the antiproteinuric effect was similar irrespective of the antihypertensive agent used.

It is of particular note that such reduction of albuminuria is seen even in normotensive microalbuminuric individuals.[40] This was shown in large studies on type 1[41] and type 2[42] diabetic patients. A consensus statement postulated that even normotensive diabetic patients should be given antihypertensive medication, preferably ACE inhibitors, irrespective of the type of diabetes. In diabetic patients such treatment of normotensive microalbuminuric patients with ACE inhibitors has the added benefit that progression of diabetic retinopathy is reduced.[43]

Selection of antihypertensive drugs for proteinuric renal disease

The large controlled prospective randomized trials on prevention of progression of renal failure in diabetic[44] or non-diabetic renal disease[39,45] were conducted with ACE inhibitors. This was based on the rationale that

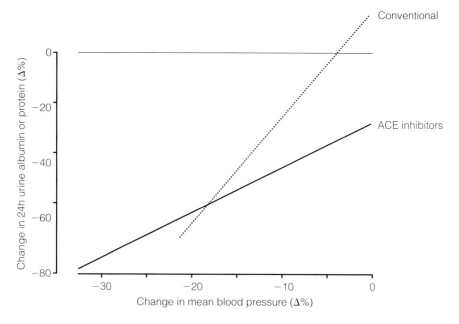

Figure 5.6

Meta-analysis of percentage changes (Δ%) in albuminuria/proteinuria as related to blood pressure changes in diabetics on ACE inhibitors or conventional diuretics and/or β-blockers. (After Weidmann et al.[39])

ACE inhibitors are superior to alternative antihypertensive agents because of their effects on glomerular hemodynamics[14] and non-hemodynamic actions.[16–18]

It is currently unresolved whether preemptive treatment with ACE inhibitors prevents the onset of microalbuminuria in diabetic individuals. The results of the EUCLID study with lisinopril clearly showed that the ACE inhibitor reduced progression of albuminuria, but the data were not entirely convincing concerning prevention of microalbuminuria. In the recent HOPE study,[46] administration of 10 mg ramipril to mostly nor-motensive individuals, amongst others, also prevented progression of microalbuminuria. It is of particular note that in several studies the reduction of cardiovascular events was particularly pronounced in patients with signs of renal dysfunction, as reflected by albuminuria/proteinuria and/or moderate elevation of S-creatinine.[47] It is not sufficiently widely known among the medical community that even a slight elevation of serum creatinine concentration is a very powerful predictor of cardiovascular risk, as shown by the Framingham, the MRFIT, the HOT[48] and the HOPE[49] studies.[49]

More recently, angiotensin II receptor-blocking (ARB) agents have been introduced. In experimental studies, they were similarly effective compared to ACE inhibitors in attenuating progression.[50] With respect to glomerular hemodynamics, important species differences have to be taken into consideration. In rats, lowering of glomerular capillary pressure is largely mediated via bradykinin and, in this respect, ACE inhibitors are superior;[51] however, there is little evidence for this in humans. With respect to short-term hemodynamic and antiproteinuric effects, Gansevoort et al.[50] showed that equipotent doses of enalapril and losartan, i.e. doses which lowered blood pressure to a similar extent, have similar effects on renal perfusion and protein excretion, as shown in *Fig. 5.7.* Currently, two large international multicenter studies in type 2 diabetic patients with advanced nephropathy are under way to assess the renoprotective effects of irbesartan and losartan: the results are expected soon. Currently, no definitive information is available.

It has recently been claimed that combination of an ACE inhibitor and an ARB is superior with respect to reducing urinary protein excretion.[51] It is very difficult to prove this point. In order to prove additive effects it is necessary to administer maximal doses of either drug, i.e. doses at the ceiling of the dose–response curve. By this definition, an additive effect has so far not been proven.

In some experimental studies, administration of CCB to animals with various models of renal damage aggravated glomerulosclerosis and proteinuria – presumably because systemic blood pressure had not been appropriately lowered.[20,21,52] Similarly, CCB – at least of the dihydropyridine type – increased proteinuria in diabetic and non-diabetic renal disease.[53] Conversely, when blood pressure was substantially lowered, some nephroprotection, i.e. lesser development of glomerulosclerosis, was seen in animals with renal damage.[17] Reduction of proteinuria was also seen in patients with renal disease, particularly in diabetic patients.[54,55] However, in experimental studies, the effect was less consistent than with ACE inhibitors and, in head-on comparisons,[56,57] it was also less pronounced. It is obvious that CCB are a very heterogenous group of agents. Whilst in type 2 diabetic patients, consistent reduction of proteinuria is seen with verapamil and diltiazem, this is not the case with nifedipine.[55] In contrast to short-acting dihydropyridine-type CCB, however, amlodipine as a long-acting dihydropyridine-type CCB was shown to have beneficial effects on proteinuria and loss of GFR. It was even equipotent with cilazepril.[58]

Based on the above, CCB should not be considered the first choice in the antihypertensive treatment of patients with renal disease, but, in clinical practice, their use is mostly indispensable because multidrug therapy is necessary in most patients in order to achieve the target blood pressures that have recently been recommended in this patient population (see below).[59] Indeed, very convincing theoretical arguments have been

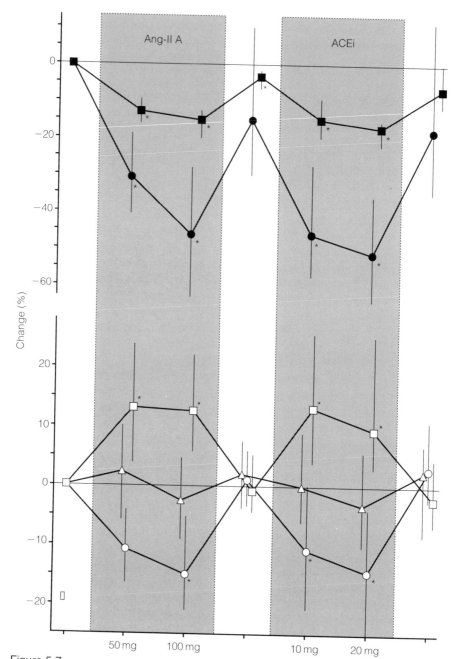

Figure 5.7

Comparison of the effects of angiotensin II (Ang-II A) receptor antagonism and ACE inhibition (ACEi). Changes in: ■, blood pressure; ●, urinary protein excretion; △, glomerular filtration rate; □, effective renal plasma flow; ○, filtration fraction; *, $p < 0.05$. (After Gansevoort et al.[50])

offered that the combination of ACE inhibitors and CCB provide particular benefit,[60] i.e. reduction of proteinuria was more pronounced with combination therapy.

Target blood pressure

In the past, it had been thought that the diseased kidney requires blood pressure values above the normal range in order to function properly. This was based on the observation that acute lowering of blood pressure may acutely reduce GFR and cause an increase in serum creatinine. These short-term effects are mainly due to disturbed renal autoregulation and are mostly reversible. In the patient with a major increase of serum creatinine after administration of ACE inhibitors, however, alternative explanations, particularly hypovolemia, mostly secondary to overzealous diuretic treatment with excessive activation of the renin–angiotensin system or the presence of undiagnosed renal artery stenosis, have to be considered.

As illustrated by several studies (see also Figs 5.4 and 5.5), it has become apparent that, in the long run, for optimal renoprotection much lower blood pressures are necessary than had been thought in the past. Based on observational studies and particularly on the results of intervention trials, such as the MDRD,[36] the REIN[38] and the UKPDS[61] studies, it has been proposed that in patients with proteinuric renal disease blood pressure should be lowered to values less than the normal values, i.e. 130/85 mmHg according to the WHO–ISH definition.[62] Table 5.1 shows the results of the UKPDS study. In this study, patients were randomized to regular or to intensified antihypertensive treatment, i.e. target blood pressures of 180/105 or 150/85 mmHg respectively.[61] This is still above what is today considered optimal, but one has to bear in mind that the study was planned when the safety of more aggressive blood pressure lowering had not been firmly established, at least in elderly diabetic

Table 5.1   Standard versus intensified blood pressure control in type 2 diabetes UKPDS[61]

Reduction of:	Risk reduction (%)
Diabetes-related end-points	24
Diabetes-related deaths	32
Strokes	44
Microvascular end-points	37

Achieved blood pressure was 144/82 or 154/87 mmHg.

patients. *Table 5.1* shows that even the modest blood pressure difference of 10 mmHg systolic and 5 mmHg diastolic had a dramatic effect on non-renal and renal outcome. As a consequence, the National Kidney Foundation[63] proposed to lower blood pressure to values as low as 125/75 mmHg in proteinuric renal disease (with excretion of >1 g protein per day).

In the past these recommendations raised concern about safety, particularly in view of the concept of the J-curve. This hypothesis implies that once blood pressure is lowered to values <85 mmHg diastolic, the rate of cardiac events increases again because coronary perfusion pressure is compromised, at least in patients with pre-existing coronary lesions. Fletcher and Bulpitt[64] provided cogent arguments that the concept of a J-curve is not tenable, although admittedly the issue is not completely settled.[65]

In this context it is important that neither a trial in non-renal patients, i.e. the HOT study,[48] nor the MDRD[36] or the UKPDS[61] trials found excess cardiovascular mortality with more aggressive blood pressure lowering. Needless to say, because of the possibility of vascular stenoses (which should be excluded by angiological studies including carotid sonography) and disturbed autoregulation (particularly in the elderly), one should lower blood pressure slowly and under careful observation of the patient.

References

1. Rettig R, Stauss H, Folberth C *et al*. Hypertension transmitted by kidneys from stroke-prone spontaneously hypertensive rats. Am J Physiol 1989; 257 (suppl F): F197–F203.

2. Curtis JJ, Luke RG, Dustan HP *et al*. Remission of essential hypertension after renal transplantation. N Engl J Med 1983; 309: 1009–1015.

3. Guyton AC. Renal function curve – a key to understanding the pathogenesis of hypertension. Hypertension 1987; 10: 1–6.

4. Koomans HA, Roos JC, Dorhout Mees EJ, Delawi IM. Sodium balance in renal failure. A comparison of patients with normal subjects under extremes of sodium intake. Hypertension 1985; 7: 714–721.

5. Harrap SB, Davies DL, Macnicol AM *et al*. Renal, cardiovascular and hormonal characteristics of young adults with autosomal dominant polycystic kidney disease. Kidney Int 1991; 40: 501–508.

6. Ritz E, Koomans HA. New insights into mechanisms of blood pressure regulation in patients with uraemia. Nephrol Dial Transpl 1996; 11: 52–59.

7. Price DA, Porter LE, Gordon M *et al*. The paradox of the low-renin state in diabetic nephropathy. J Am Soc Nephrol 1999; 10: 2382–2391.

8. Converse RL Jr, Jacobsen TN, Toto RD *et al*. Sympathetic overactivity in patients with chronic renal failure. N Engl J Med 1992; 327: 1912–1918.

9. Campese VM, Kogosov E. Renal

afferent denervation prevents hypertension in rats with chronic renal failure. Hypertension 1995; 25: 878–882.

10. Amann K, Rump LC, Simonaviciene A et al. Effects of low dose sympathetic inhibition on glomerulosclerosis and albuminuria in subtotally nephrectomized rats. J Am Soc Nephrol 2000; 11: 1469–1478.

11. Strojek K, Grzeszczak W, Gorska J, Leschinger MI, Ritz E. Lowering of microalbuminuria in diabetic patients by a sympathicoplegic agent: novel approach to prevent progression of diabetic nephropathy? J Am Soc Nephrol 2001; 12: 602–605.

12. Bidani AK, Mitchell KD, Schwartz MM et al. Absence of glomerular injury or nephron loss in a normotensive rat remnant kidney model. Kidney Int 1990; 38: 28–38.

13. Gloy J, Henger A, Fischer KG et al. Angiotensin II modulates cellular functions of podocytes. Kidney Int 1998; 67 (suppl): S168–S170.

14. Anderson S, Rennke HG, Brenner BM. Therapeutic advantage of converting enzyme inhibitors in arresting progressive renal disease associated with systemic hypertension in the rat. J Clin Invest 1986; 77: 1993–2000.

15. Griffin KA, Picken M, Bidani AK. Radiotelemetric BP monitoring, antihypertensives and glomeruloprotection in remnant kidney model. Kidney Int 1994; 46: 1010–1018.

16. Amann K, Irzyniec T, Mall G, Ritz E. The effect of enalapril on glomerular growth and glomerular lesions after subtotal nephrectomy in the rat: a stereological analysis. J Hypertens 1993; 11: 969–975.

17. Tolins JP, Raij L. Comparison of converting enzyme inhibitor and calcium channel blocker in hypertensive glomerular injury. Hypertension 1990; 16: 452–61.

18. Remuzzi A, Imberti O, Puntorieri S et al. Dissociation between antiproteinuric and antihypertensive effect of angiotensin converting enzyme inhibitors in rats. Am J Physiol 1994; 267 (suppl F): F1034–F1044.

19. Peters H, Border WA, Noble NA. Targeting TGF-beta overexpression in renal disease: maximizing the antifibrotic action of angiotensin II blockade. Kidney Int 1998; 54: 1570–1580.

20. Brunner FP, Thiel G, Hermle M et al. Long-term enalapril and verapamil in rats with reduced renal mass. Kidney Int 1989; 36: 969–977.

21. Wenzel UO, Troschau G, Schoeppe W et al. Adverse effect of the calcium channel blocker nitrendipine on nephrosclerosis in rats with renovascular hypertension. Hypertension 1992; 20: 233–241.

22. Reams GP, Villarreal D, Wu Z et al. An evaluation of the renal protective effect of manidipine in the uninephrectomized spontaneously hypertensive rat. Am Heart J 1995; 125: 620–625.

23. Dworkin LD, Levin RI, Benstein JA et al. Effects of nifedipine and enalapril on glomerular injury in rats with deoxycorticosterone-salt hypertension. Am J Physiol 1990; 259 (suppl F): F578–F604.

24. Irzyniec T, Mall G, Greber D, Ritz E. Beneficial effect of nifedipine and moxonidine on glomerulosclerosis in spontaneously hypertensive rats. A micromorphometric study. Am J Hypertens 1992; 5: 437–443.

25. Mitch WE, Walser M, Buffington GA, Lemann J Jr. A simple method of estimating progression of chronic renal failure. Lancet 1976; 2: 1326–1328.

26. Mogensen CE. Systemic blood pressure and glomerular leakage with particular reference to diabetes and hypertension. J Intern Med 1994; 235: 297–316.

27. Parving HH. Impact of blood pressure and antihypertensive treatment on incipient and overt nephropathy, retinopathy, and endothelial permeability in diabetes mellitus. Diabetes Care 1991; 14: 260–269.

28. Brazy PC, Stead WW, Fitzwilliam JF. Progression of renal insufficiency: role of blood pressure. Kidney Int 1989; 35: 670–674.

29. Hannedouche T, Albouze G, Chauveau P et al. Effects of blood pressure and antihypertensive treatment on progression of advanced chronic renal failure. Am J Kidney Dis 1993; 21: 131–137.

30. Opelz G, Wujciak T, Ritz E. Association of chronic kidney graft failure with recipient blood pressure. Collaborative Transplant Study. Kidney Int 1998; 53: 217–222.

31. Timio M, Venanzi S, Lolli S et al. 'Non-dipper' hypertensive patients and progressive renal insufficiency: a 3-year longitudinal study. Clin Nephrol 1995; 43: 382–387.

32. Farmer CK, Goldsmith DJ, Quin JD et al. Progression of diabetic nephropathy – is diurnal blood pressure rhythm as important as absolute blood pressure level? Nephrol Dial Transplant 1998; 13: 635–639.

33. Mogensen CE. In: Andreucci VE, Fine LG, eds. International Yearbook of Nephrology. Springer: London, 1995, 141.

34. Nielsen FS, Rossing P, Gall MA et al. Long-term effect of lisinopril and atenolol on kidney function in hypertensive NIDDM subjects with diabetic nephropathy. Diabetes 1997; 46: 1182–1188.

35. Apperloo AJ, de Zeeuw D, de Jong PE. A short-term antihypertensive treatment-induced fall in glomerular filtration rate predicts long-term stability of renal function. Kidney Int 1997; 51: 793–797.

36. Klahr S, Levey AS, Beck GJ et al. The effects of dietary protein restriction and blood-pressure control on the progression of chronic renal disease. Modification of Diet in Renal Disease Study Group. N Engl J Med 1994; 330: 877–884.

37. Maschio G, Alberti D, Janin G et al. Effect of the angiotensin-converting-enzyme inhibitor benazepril on the progression of chronic renal insufficiency. The Angiotensin-Converting-Enzyme Inhibition in Progressive Renal Insufficiency Study Group. N Engl J Med 1996; 334: 939–945.

38. The GISEN Group (Gruppo Italiano di Studi Epidemiologici in Nefrologia). Randomised placebo-controlled trial of effect of ramipril on decline in glomerular filtration rate and risk of terminal renal failure in proteinuric, non-diabetic nephropathy. Lancet 1997; 349: 1857–1863.

39. Weidmann P, Schneider M, Bohlen L. Therapeutic efficacy of different antihypertensive drugs in human diabetic nephropathy: an updated meta-analysis. Nephrol Dial Transplant 1995; 10 (suppl 9): 39–45.

40. Mogensen CE, Keane WF, Bennett PH et al. Prevention of diabetic renal disease with special reference to microalbuminuria. Lancet 1995; 346: 1080–1084.

41. Viberti G, Mogensen CE, Groop LC, Pauls JF. Effect of captopril on progression to clinical proteinuria in patients with insulin-dependent diabetes mellitus and microalbuminuria. European Micro-

albuminuria Captopril Study Group. JAMA 1994; 271: 275–279.

42. Ravid M, Brosh D, Levi Z *et al.* Use of enalapril to attenuate decline in renal function in normotensive, normoalbuminuric patients with type 2 diabetes mellitus. A randomized, controlled trial. Ann Intern Med 1998; 128: 982–988.

43. Chaturvedi N, Sjolie AK, Stephenson JM *et al.* Effect of lisinopril on progression of retinopathy in normotensive people with type 1 diabetes. The EUCLID Study Group. EURODIAB Controlled Trial of Lisinopril in Insulin-Dependent Diabetes Mellitus. Lancet 1998; 351: 28–31.

44. Lewis EJ, Hunsicker LG, Bain RP, Rohde RD. The effect of angiotensin-converting-enzyme inhibition on diabetic nephropathy. The Collaborative Study Group. N Engl J Med 1993; 329: 1456–1462.

45. Maschio G, Alberti D, Janin G *et al.* Effect of the angiotensin-converting-enzyme inhibitor benazepril on the progression of chronic renal insufficiency. The Angiotensin-Converting-Enzyme Inhibition in Progressive Renal Insufficiency Study Group. N Engl J Med 1996; 334: 939–945.

46. Chaturvedi N. HOPE and extension of the indications for ACE inhibitors? Heart Outcomes Prevention Evaluation. Lancet 2000; 355: 246–247.

47. Rouilope LM, Salvetti A, Jamerson K *et al.* Renal function and intensive lowering of blood pressure in hypertensive participants of the hypertension optimal treatment (HOT) study. J Am Soc Nephrol 2001; 12: 218–225.

48. Hansson L, Zanchetti A, Carruthers SG *et al.* Effects of intensive blood-pressure lowering and low-dose aspirin in patients with hypertension: principal results of the Hypertension Optimal Treatment (HOT) randomised trial. HOT Study Group. Lancet 1998; 351: 1755–1762.

49. Mann JFE. Should the results of the HOPE study affect the nephrological practice? Nephrol Dial Transplant 2000; 15: 453–54.

50. Gansevoort RT, de Zeeuw D, de Jong PE. Is the antiproteinuric effect of ACE inhibition mediated by interference in the renin-angiotensin system? Kidney Int 1994; 45: 861–867.

51. Russo D, Pisani A, Balletta MM *et al.* Additive antiproteinuric effect of converting enzyme inhibitor and losartan in normotensive patients with IgA nephropathy. Am J Kidney Dis 1999; 33: 851–856.

52. Brunner FP, Bock HA, Hermle M *et al.* Control of hypertension by verapamil enhances renal damage in a rat remnant kidney model. Nephrol Dial Transplant 1991; 420–427.

53. Kloke HJ, Wetzels JF, Koene RA, Huysmans FT. Effects of low-dose nifedipine on urinary protein excretion rate in patients with renal disease. Nephrol Dial Transplant 1998; 13: 646–650.

54. Bakris GL. Effects of diltiazem or lisinopril on massive proteinuria associated with diabetes mellitus. Ann Intern Med 1990; 112: 707–708.

55. Bakris GL, Barnhill BW, Sadler R. Treatment of arterial hypertension in diabetic humans: importance of therapeutic selection. Kidney Int 1992; 41: 912–919.

56. Jackson B, Johnston CI. The contribution of systemic hypertension to progression of chronic renal failure in the rat remnant kidney: effect of treatment with an angiotensin converting enzyme

inhibitor or a calcium inhibitor. J Hypertens 1988; 6: 495–501.

57. Perico N, Amuchastegui CS, Malanchini B *et al.* Angiotensin-converting-enzyme inhibition and calcium channel blockade both normalize early hyperfiltration in experimental diabetes, but only the former prevents late renal structural damage. Exp Nephrol 1994; 2: 220–228.

58. Velussi M, Brocco E, Frigato F *et al.* Effects of cilazapril and amlodipine on kidney function in hypertensive NIDDM patients. Diabetes 1996; 45: 216–222.

59. Schwenger V, Ritz E. Audit of antihypertensive treatment in patients with renal failure. Nephrol Dial Transplant 1998; 13: 3091–3095.

60. Bakris GI, Weir M, DeQuattro V *et al.* Renal hemodynamic and antiproteinuric response to an ACE inhibitor, trandolapril, or calcium antagonist, verapamil alone or in fixed dose combination in patients with diabetic nephropathy – a randomised multicenter study. J Am Soc Nephrol 1996; 7: 1546A.

61. UK Prospective Diabetes Study Group (UKPDS). Tight blood pressure control and risk of macrovascular and microvascular complications in type 2 diabetes: UKPDS 38. BMJ 1998; 317: 703–713.

62. World Health Organization–International Society of Hypertension (WHO–ISH). WHO–ISH Guidelines for the Management of Hypertension. Guidelines Subcommittee. J Hypertens 1999; 17: 151–183.

63. Jacobson HR, Striker GE. Report on a workshop to develop management recommendations for the prevention of progression in chronic renal disease. Am J Kidney Dis 1995; 25: 103–106.

64. Fletcher AE, Bulpitt CJ. How far should blood pressure be lowered? N Engl J Med 1992; 326: 251–254.

65. Kaplan N. J-curve not burned off by HOT study. Hypertension Optimal Treatment. Lancet 1998; 351: 1748–1749.

6
Management of hypertension in diabetic patients

Norman M Kaplan

Introduction

Largely as a consequence of obesity, hypertension and diabetes frequently coexist. On the one hand, hypertension is found in >70% of all diabetics and about 75% of cardiovascular disease (CVD) in diabetes is attributable to the coexisting hypertension.[1] On the other hand, the risk for developing diabetes is almost doubled by the presence of hypertension even among non-obese people with blood pressure only as high as 130/85 mmHg.[2] When the two coexist, cardiovascular–renal complications occur at a much higher rate, at least two-fold overall and many fold for progressive nephropathy.[1]

There may be an obvious explanation for some of the increased prevalence of hypertension, nephropathy, and diabetes: hyperglycemia during pregnancy reduces nephrogenesis in the fetus.[3] Just as maternal protein deprivation leads to a reduced number of nephrons, so could hyperglycemia. The infants of women with abnormal glucose tolerance or overt diabetes would then be susceptible to more hypertension, diabetes, and nephropathy.

Beyond the possible contribution of impaired fetal development, there are a number of other reasons for the increasing prevalence of diabetes and hypertension. These include:

(a) advancing age of the population;
(b) increasing prevalence of obesity due to decreased physical inactivity and increased caloric intake;
(c) prolonged survival of type 1 diabetic patients;
(d) expanding reach of medical care.

Predominant role of obesity

Obesity is increasing in all industrialized societies and the current US population is likely the fattest of all time. Obesity, defined as a body mass index (BMI) >30 kg/m^2, increased from 12% of US adults in 1991 to 17.9% in 1998.[4] The increase occurred in virtually every part of the population, among men and women, from the teens to old age, in all races and socio-economic strata.

With increasing BMI, the incidence of type 2 diabetes increases markedly. A 5 kg weight gain doubles the risk for diabetes and risk increases with the duration of excess weight.[5] The problem begins in early childhood, where increasing weight is associated with hyperinsulinemia and increasing blood pressure and dyslipidemia, particularly in those with greater central (visceral or abdominal) obesity,[6] the components of the metabolic syndrome.

Obviously, greater attention must be given to those who are both diabetic and hypertensive: in a recent European survey, only about 11% of type 1 diabetic patients had their hypertension adequately controlled.[7]

Increasing recognition of the problem

All three recently published guidelines from expert committees have emphasized the need both for earlier intervention at even lower levels of blood pressure for hypertensives with diabetes and for more intensive therapy.

(a) JNC VI places all diabetics in the highest risk category (group C), wherein immediate drug therapy is indicated if blood pressure is >130/85 mmHg.[8]
(b) WHO–ISH places all diabetics with blood pressure >140/90 mmHg into risk group III (high risk), with a 15–20% risk of a major cardiovascular event over the next 10 years; those with blood pressure >180/110 mmHg are in risk group IV (very high risk) with >30% risk over 10 years.[9] Drug therapy is recommended immediately for both groups.
(c) The British Hypertension Society recommends that drug treatment be started in those with a blood pressure >140/90 mmHg, with a target of <140/80 mmHg.[10]

Assessment of blood pressure

Before therapy is begun, the presence of usually elevated blood pressure must be carefully ascertained. Such ascertainment should include out-of-the-office readings. As with all patients, out-of-the-office measurements are needed both to establish the diagnosis and to monitor the management. White-coat hypertension is common, particularly among young type 1 diabetics and, if not recognized, may lead to misdiagnosis.[11]

Ambulatory blood pressure monitoring (ABPM) is the best technique to recognize white-coat hypertension. With ABPM, the common lack of nocturnal dipping in diabetics can be recognized and should lead to more intensive control of the blood pressure.[11]

Recognition of postural hypotension

All diabetics, particularly if over the age of 60, should have their blood pressure measured supine and standing, since postural and postprandial hypotension is common and potentially hazardous. In 204 type 2 diabetics, average age of 58, postural hypotension was found in 28.4% and postural dizziness in 22.5%.[12] If present, postural and postprandial hypotension must be managed before supine and seated hypertension is treated.

Non-pharmacological therapy

Therapy for all hypertension should begin and continue with lifestyle modifications, even more so in the typically obese type 2 diabetic (*Table 6.1*). Despite the obvious attraction of lifestyle changes, they are hard to accomplish and may not be as protective as drug therapy. The high risk of hypertension with type 2 diabetes almost mandates early and intensive antihypertensive drug therapy.

Weight loss

Weight loss lowers blood pressure at least in part by improving insulin sensitivity.[13] The value of weight loss was documented by the impressive reduction in the cumulative incidence of overt diabetes seen in a randomized trial of weight reduction in 522 overweight subjects who had abnormal glucose tolerance.[14] Diabetes developed in 23% of the control group but in only 11% of those who lost an average of 3.5 kg by diet and physical activity.

Table 6.1   Lifestyle modifications for hypertension

Stop smoking
Lose weight if overweight
Reduce sodium intake to 110 mmol per day (2.4 g sodium or 6 g sodium chloride)
Maintain adequate dietary potassium, calcium, and magnesium intake
Increase physical activity
Limit alcohol intake to ≤1 oz per day of ethanol (24 oz of beer, 8 oz of wine, or 2 oz of 100-proof whiskey)

Exercise

Those who are sedentary and unfit develop more diabetes whether lean or obese. Just walking, without more vigorous activity, reduces the risk for diabetes and will lower blood pressure.[15] The manner by which exercise helps both diabetes and hypertension goes beyond a decrease in body weight. Exercise increases glucose uptake into skeletal muscles, making them more insulin sensitive. The benefits of exercise in patients with diabetes include improvement in glycemic control, lowering of blood pressure, reduction in levels of triglyceride-rich very low-density lipoproteins (VLDL), probable improvement in fibrinolytic activity, and reduction in CVD.

Moderate sodium reduction

Moderate sodium reduction is both safe and effective,[16] perhaps even more in those diabetics whose hypertension is related to volume expansion from renal impairment. Moreover, the antiproteinuric effect of angiotensin-converting-enzyme (ACE) inhibitors is markedly enhanced by a lower sodium intake.[17] But even without nephropathy, diabetic patients need to reduce their sodium intake since insulin-resistant subjects have an impaired natriuretic response to high sodium intake.[18]

The value of moderate sodium reduction was shown in 34 type 2 diabetic hypertensives wherein a reduction of sodium intake of 60 mmol per day for 3 months was associated with a 20 mmHg fall in systolic pressure; when sodium intake was increased, the blood pressure rose by 11 mmHg.[19]

Moderate alcohol consumption

Diabetics have been found to obtain a protective effect against coronary disease by regular, moderate alcohol consumption (no more than two drinks a day) similar to that seen in multiple other groups.[20] In addition to multiple other mechanisms for the cardioprotection provided by moderate amounts of alcohol, insulin sensitivity is improved.[21] In turn, the risk of developing type 2 diabetes was reduced by 42% among middle-aged Japanese men who drank moderately.[22]

The type of alcoholic beverage is likely irrelevant: wine drinkers have the lowest risk for coronary disease, likely because of their healthier lifestyle; red wine drinkers have no greater protection than white wine drinkers.[23]

Cessation of smoking

As the most important lifestyle to be addressed, smoking may also markedly aggravate insulin resistance in type 2 diabetics.[24]

Dietary fiber

In a large population of young, healthy subjects, increased dietary fiber intake was associated with lower body weight, lower waist-to-hip ratio, lower fasting insulin, lower blood pressure, and better lipid profiles.[25]

Antihypertensive drug therapy

The protective effect of antihypertensive therapy in diabetic hypertensives has been well documented, with all four of the major classes of drugs – low-dose diuretics, β-blockers, ACE inhibitors and calcium-channel blockers (CCB).[26]

The best documentation of the need to lower diastolic blood pressure ≤80 mmHg in diabetic hypertensives comes from the Hypertension Optimal Treatment (HOT) trial.[27] Among the 19,000 participants in the trial, the only significant benefit of reducing the diastolic blood pressure to near 80 mmHg was seen among the 1501 diabetic hypertensives. They achieved >50% reduction in major cardiovascular events (*Fig. 6.1*). As found in the HOT trial, to achieve the necessary goal of blood pressure <130/80 mmHg, two or more antihypertensive drugs will usually be needed.

Further evidence for the need for more intensive therapy comes from the population of 3642 type 2 diabetics screened for the United Kingdom

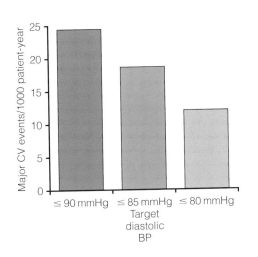

Figure 6.1

The risk for major cardiovascular (CV) events in the 1501 diabetic patients in the Hypertension Optimal Treatment (HOT) study according to the fertile of the target diastolic blood pressure (BP) level. $p < 0.005$ for trend (n = 1501). (Adapted from Hansson *et al.*[27])

Prospective Diabetes Study (UKPDS) but not entered into the trial.[28] A progressive reduction in major cardiovascular events was seen, with progressive reduction of systolic blood pressure from > 160 mmHg down to 100 mmHg as provided by various antihypertensive drugs.[28]

To provide the other essential corrections for concomitant risk factors, multiple non-drug and drug therapies will be needed: the benefits of such intensive therapy are impressive.[29] In this trial by Gaede et al.,[29] 160 diabetics with microalbuminuria were randomly assigned to standard or more intensive therapy, the latter requiring a blood pressure < 140/85 mmHg, Hemoglobin $A1_C$ (HbA1$_C$) < 6.5%, total cholesterol < 5 mmol/l, and the use of ACE inhibitors, aspirin plus multiple lifestyle modifications. At the end of the 3.8 years follow-up, those on intensive therapy achieved major benefits (*Fig. 6.2*). Such intensive therapies, though costly, will not only reduce morbidity and mortality but also lower lifetime medical costs.

Choice of antihypertensive drugs

For those diabetic hypertensives without proteinuria, a low-dose diuretic may be the appropriate first choice with an ACE inhibitor (ACEI) as second drug and a long-acting CCB as third. Both β-blockers and α-blockers may be indicated. Rarely, central $α_2$-agonists may be useful. For those with proteinuria, an ACEI is mandatory. An angitensin II receptor blocker (ARB) should be substituted if a cough precludes use of an ACEI and may become the initial choice in view of recently reported, but still unpublished, data from three clinical trials in type 2 diabetics with nephropathy, wherein excellent renal protection was seen.

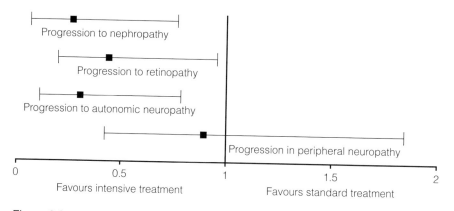

Figure 6.2

The development or progression of microvascular complications in the 80 diabetic hypertensives assigned to standard treatment compared to the 80 patients assigned to intensive treatment. (Reprinted with permission from Gaede et al.[29].)

Diuretics

Low doses, i.e. 12.5 mg of hydrochlorothiazide, are effective and safe in diabetics, as shown in the Systolic Hypertension in the Elderly Program (SHEP) trial.[30] A thiazide diuretic should be almost always included in the regimen and loop diuretics given to those with serum creatinine >1.5 mg/dl.

β-Blockers

Despite many warnings about their potential to aggravate diabetes in various ways, β-blockers may be effective and safe. They are mandatory for those who survive a myocardial infarction.[8] Since they were somewhat more protective than an ACEI in the UKPDS trial,[31] their use may increase.

α-Blockers

In addition to their ability to relieve prostatism, α-blockers are better than any other class in reducing insulin resistance and improving dyslipidemia. When used alone in high-risk patients, such as those enrolled in the Antihypertensive and Lipid-Lowering Treatment to Prevent Heart Attack (ALLHAT) trial,[32] they may expose the patient to congestive heart failure.[33] Therefore, they should always be given with a low-dose diuretic.

CCB

Concerns have been expressed about the safety of CCB, particularly the dihydropyridines (DHP) and especially in diabetic hypertensives. As to their putative effect to increase coronary disease, the problem remains unique to large doses of short-acting agents and does not apply to long-acting agents. The safety of long-acting CCB in patients with coronary disease was further documented in a 1 year follow-up of over 51,000 patients who were prescribed one of these agents after surviving an acute myocardial infarction.[34] Their relative likelihood of 1-year mortality was no different than among those not prescribed a long-acting CCB.

As to their particular effects in diabetes, most of the current evidence of a benefit from antihypertensive therapy in diabetics comes from trials using DHP CCB. Birkenhager and Staessen[35] defend the use of DHP–CCB in diabetic hypertensives as follows:

(a) the excellent protection found in the Systolic Hypertension in Europe (Syst-Eur) trial with nitrendipine, even better than that found in a similar group of hypertensive diabetics given a diuretic in the SHEP trial;[36]

Table 6.2   Studies reporting outcome in diabetic patients with
hypertension

Study	Diabetic patients n (%)*	Main study drugs
Placebo-controlled trials		
SHEP	590 (12.3)	Chlorthalidone[†] versus placebo
Syst-China	98 (4.1)	Nitrendipine[†] versus placebo
Syst-Eur	492 (10.5)	Nitrendipine[†] versus placebo
Trials other than placebo-controlled		
ABCD	470 (100)[‡]	Nisoldipine versus enalapril[†]
ALLHAT	40,000 (± 33)	Amlodipine or lisinopril versus chlorthalidone (still ongoing)
FACET	380 (100)	Amlodipine versus fosinopril[†]
HOT	1501 (8.0)	Felodipine to reach diastolic BP ≤90 mmHg[†] or ≤80 mmHg
UKPDS	1148 (100)	Atenolol or captopril to reach BP <150/85 mmHg[†] or <180/105 mmHg

*Number of diabetic patients (percentage of total number of patients enrolled); † with this treatment, outcome was significantly better in diabetic patients with hypertension; ‡ results in 480 normotensive diabetic patients were not reported.
ABCD, Appropriate Blood Pressure Control in Diabetes; ALLHAT, Antihypertensive and Lipid Lowering Treatment to Prevent Heart Attack Trial; FACET, Fosinopril versus Amlodipine Cardiovascular Events Trial; HOT, Hypertension Optimal Treatment; SHEP, Systolic Hypertension in the Elderly Program; Syst-China, Systolic Hypertension in China; Syst-Eur, Systolic Hypertension in Europe; UKPDS, United Kingdom Prospective Diabetes Study.

(b) the major reduction in cardiovascular events in the 1501 diabetics given felodipine-based therapy in the HOT trial (See *Fig. 6.1*);[27]
(c) the presumed lack of significant adverse effects in the amlodipine quarter of the ongoing ALLHAT trial with over 15,000 diabetics enrolled,[32] since the Safety Monitoring Committee has not called for a discontinuation of the amlodipine limb of the trial, now in its fifth year.

Additional evidence in defense of the benefits of CCB for treatment of hypertensive diabetics comes from the results of the 719 diabetics among the 6614 elderly hypertensives in the Swedish Trial of Old Persons with Hypertension-2 (STOP-Hypertension-2) study, the only completed trial that compares drugs from the three major classes, i.e. diuretics/β-blockers, ACEI and CCB.[37] A lower rate of coronary heart disease and heart failure was seen in those taking an ACEI, but a lower rate of stroke and mortality in those on a CCB.

The data now available provide no clear evidence that one class of drug is superior, although in all of the comparative trials of diabetic

Table 6.3   Rates of events per 1000 patients in the seven comparative trials in diabetic hypertensives

	No. points	Total events per 1000 patients*			
		CHD	CHF	Stroke	Mortality
Diuretic and/or β-blocker	1903	75	27	62	125
ACEI†	1368	87	32	66	121
CCB‡	1657	71	32	53	83

*CHD, coronary heart disease; CHF, coronary heart failure; † angiotensin-converting-enzyme inhibitor; ‡ calcium-channel blocker.

hypertensives, CCB-based therapy has been associated with fewer events than either diuretic- or ACEI-based therapy (*Table 6.3*).[38]

The bottom line, at present, is that either DHP or non-DHP CCB are frequently needed to control the hypertension in most diabetics, particularly to prevent the progression of renal damage. They may be renoprotective even if they do not reduce proteinuria. In a 42+ month follow-up of 48 proteinuric diabetics, the half given a DHP CCB, nisoldipine, had no reduction in proteinuria but a lesser fall in glomerular filtration rate (GFR) than did the half given an ACEI.[39]

ACEI

An ACEI should always be used for those with proteinuria. This is likely to be expanded to normotensive diabetics with microalbuminuria: over 4 years, nine of 23 such patients on placebo advanced to diabetic nephropathy, whereas only two of 21 given captopril advanced.[40]

Whether an ACEI should also be the routine first drug for all diabetics without microalbuminuria is less certain, but is looking more and more likely. In the Captopril Prevention Project (CAPPP), those diabetics given captopril had fewer events than did those given diuretics and β-blockers, whereas there was no difference in the non-diabetics.[41] On the other hand, the ACEI was somewhat less protective than the β-blocker in the UKPDS trial, the largest and longest trial involving type 2 diabetic hypertensives.[31]

The renin–angiotensin system may be set inappropriately higher in type 2 diabetics so that there is a theoretical reason to use ACEI. Certainly, ACEI have been found to be protective in diabetic patients who have survived a myocardial infarction.[42] In the Heart Outcomes Prevention Evaluation (HOPE) trial, the 9297 patients with known CVD included 38% with diabetes; over the 4–6 year follow-up, a 17% risk reduction for diabetic complications was reported for those given the ACEI ramapril compared to those assigned to placebo.[43]

Attractive as they are, ACEI may cause problems. They increase the risk of hypoglycemia and hyperkalemia, and may worsen renal function in those with unrecognized bilateral renovascular disease.

ARB

For the 10% of patients given an ACEI who develop a cough, an ARB is a logical alternative. Their more widespread usage is not recommended in any of the three recent guidelines[8-10] but they are being widely promoted for initial therapy. In view of the protective effect of ARB in three controlled trials – IDNT, IRMA, and RENAAL – their use will likely increase in patients with type 2 diabetes and nephropathy.

These agents are in many ways similar to ACEI but the renin–angiotensin system has three features that may give rise to differences in the benefits of ARB versus ACEI.

(a) Non-ACE alternative pathways for generation of angiotensin II have been recognized. In particular, the chymotrypsin-like serine protease chymase has been found in heart tissue and is shown to have the ability to convert AI to AII, even in the presence of natural protease inhibitors.[44]

(b) Beneficial effects of the increased levels of bradykinin that accompany ACEI but not ARB have been observed. These include:
  (i)   adding to the antihypertensive effect of ACEI;
  (ii) providing an important vasodilation that is mediated by nitric oxide.
  (iii) inhibiting vascular smooth muscle cell growth.

(c) Activation of the AT_2 receptors: most of the adverse effects of the renin–angiotensin system are mediated through the AT_1 receptor, but increasing evidence supports beneficial effects mediated through the AT_2 receptor. Initial concerns that the increased levels of AII that circulate when the AT_1 receptor is blocked could induce deleterious effects have been largely replaced with evidence that AT_2 receptor stimulation is likely beneficial. For example, overexpression of AT_2 receptor activates the vascular kinin system and causes vasodilation.[45]

Clinical effects of ARB

The multiple ARB now available seem equipotent and equally free of side effects, although angioedema has been noted with their use.[46] Losartan appears to be unique in having a modest uricosuric effect.

ARB reverse left ventricular hypertrophy and diminish proteinuria. The only published outcome study comparing an ARB versus an ACEI, the

ELITE II trial in patients with heart failure, found no difference.[47] As noted, data from three trials showing benefits of ARB in type 2 diabetics with nephropathy will soon be available.

Potential for additive effects
Since the two classes of ARB have different effects on various parts of the renin–angiotensin system, an additive effect may occur when they are used together. Preliminary evidence has been reported for additive effects of the combination of low doses of lisinopril and losartan on blood pressure,[48] and of candesartan and lisinopril on both blood pressure and microalbuminuria.[49]

Other drugs for hypertensive diabetics

Antidiabetic agents

In addition to chronic effects, hyperglycemia will acutely raise blood pressure, probably by activating the renin system. To achieve adequate glycemic control, most patients will require multiple therapies. There may be special vasodilatory effects of glitazones mediated through increased nitric oxide synthesis.[50] Any therapy that improves insulin sensitivity or lowers insulinemia should have long-term vascular protective effects.

Statins

The 483 diabetics in the Scandinavian Simvastatin Survival Study showed as much benefit as the remainder of the subjects.[51] Even though statins may not improve insulin sensitivity, they have vasodilatory effects that may be additive to those provided by ACEI.

Conclusions

Hypertension and diabetes commonly coexist and post a serious threat. Fortunately, significant protection can be provided but the benefits may be hard to achieve. Often, three or more antihypertensive drugs are needed to reach the appropriate goal of therapy, i.e. a blood pressure <130/85 mmHg.[52] Nonetheless, more intensive therapy for this rapidly expanding, highly vulnerable, population is clearly needed.

References

1. Sowers JR, Epstein M, Frohlich ED. Diabetes, hypertension, and cardiovascular disease. Hypertension 2001; 37: 1053–1059.

2. Hayashi T, Tsumura K, Suematsu C et al. High normal blood pressure, hypertension and the risk of type 2 diabetes in Japanese men. Diabetes Care 1999; 22: 1683–1687.

3. Amri K, Freund N, Vilar J et al. Adverse effects of hyperglycemia on kidney development in rats. Diabetes 1999; 48: 2240–2245.

4. Mokdad AH, Serdula MK, Dietz WH et al. The spread of the obesity epidemic in the United States, 1991–1998. JAMA 1999; 282: 1519–1522.

5. Wannamethee SG, Shaper AG. Weight change and duration of overweight and obesity in the incidence of type 2 diabetes. Diabetes Care 1999; 22: 1266–1272.

6. Morrison JA, Sprecher DL, Barton BA et al. Overweight, fat patterning, and cardiovascular disease risk factors in black and white girls: the National Heart, Lung, and Blood Institute Growth and Health Study. J Pediatr 1999; 135: 458–464.

7. Collado-Mesa F, Colhoun HM, Stevens LK et al. Prevalence and management of hypertension in type 1 diabetes mellitus in Europe: the EURODIAB IDDM Complications Study. Diabetic Med 1999; 16: 41–48.

8. Joint National Committee. The sixth report of the Joint National Committee on Prevention, Detection, Evaluation and Treatment of High Blood Pressure. Arch Intern Med 1997; 157: 2413–2446.

9. Guidelines Subcommittee. World Health Organization–International Society of Hypertension Guidelines for the Management of Hypertension. Hypertension 1999; 17: 151–183.

10. Ramsay LE, Williams B, Johnston GD et al. British Hypertension Society guidelines for hypertension management 1999: summary. BMJ 1999; 319: 630–635.

11. Holl RW, Pavlovic M, Heinze E, Thon A. Circadian blood pressure during the early course of type 1 diabetes. Diabetes Care 1999; 22: 1151–1157.

12. Wu J-S, Lu F-H, Yang Y-C, Chang C-J. postural hypotension and postural dizziness in patients with non-insulin dependent diabetes. Arch Intern Med 1999; 159: 1350–1356.

13. Ikeda T, Gomi T, Hirawa N, Sakurai JNY. Improvement of insulin sensitivity contributes to blood pressure reduction after weight loss in hypertensive subjects with obesity. Hypertension 1996; 27: 1180–1186.

14. Tuomilehto J, Lindström J, Eriksson JG et al. Prevention of type 2 diabetes mellitus by changes in lifestyle among subjects with impaired glucose tolerance. N Engl J Med 2001; 344: 1343–1350.

15. Hu FB, Sigal RJ, Rich-Edwards JW et al. Walking compared with vigorous physical activity and risk of type 2 diabetes in women. JAMA 1999; 282: 1433–1439.

16. He J, Ogden LG, Vupputuri S et al. Dietary sodium intake and subsequent risk of cardiovascular disease in overweight adults. JAMA 1999; 282: 2027–2034.

17. Buter H, Hemmelder MH, Navis G et al. The blunting of the antiproteinuric efficacy of ACE inhibition by high sodium intake can be restored by hydrochlorothiazide.

Nephrol Dial Transplant 1998; 13: 1682–1685.

18. Facchini FS, DoNascimento C, Reaven GM *et al.* Blood pressure, sodium intake, insulin resistance and urinary nitrate excretion. Hypertension 1999; 33: 1008–1012.

19. Dodson PM, Beevers M, Hallworth R *et al.* Sodium restriction and blood pressure in hypertensive type II diabetics: randomised blind controlled and crossover studies of moderate sodium restriction and sodium supplementation. BMJ 1989; 298: 227–230.

20. Valmadrid CT, Klein R, Moss SE *et al.* Alcohol intake and the risk of coronary heart disease mortality in persons with older-onset diabetes mellitus. JAMA 1999; 282: 239–246.

21. Kiechl S, Willeit J, Poewe W *et al.* Insulin sensitivity and regular alcohol consumption: large, prospective, cross sectional population study (Bruneck study). BMJ 1996; 313: 1040–1044.

22. Tsumura K, Hayashi T, Suematsu C *et al.* Daily alcohol consumption and the risk of type 2 diabetes in Japanese men. Diabetes Care 1999; 22: 1432–1437.

23. Klatsky AL, Armstrong MA, Friedman GD. Red wine, white wine, liquor, beer, and risk for coronary artery disease hospitalization. Am J Cardiol 1997; 80: 416–420.

24. Targher G, Alberiche M, Zenere MB *et al.* Cigarette smoking and insulin resistance in patients with non insulin-dependent diabetes mellitus. J Clin Endocr Metab 1997; 82: 3619–3624.

25. Ludwig DS, Pereira MA, Kroenke CH *et al.* Dietary fiber, weight gain, and cardiovascular disease risk factors in young adults. JAMA 1999; 282: 1539–1546.

26. Messerli FH, Grossman E, Goldbourt U. Antihypertensive therapy in diabetic hypertensive patients. Am J Hypertens 2001; 14: 12S–16S.

27. Hansson L, Zanchetti A, Carruthers SG *et al.* Effects of intensive blood-pressure lowering and low-dose aspirin in patients with hypertension: principal results of the Hypertension Optimal Treatment (HOT) randomised trial. Lancet 1998; 351: 1755–1762.

28. Adler AI, Stratton IM, Neill HAW *et al.* Association of systolic blood pressure with macrovascular and microvascular complications of type 2 diabetes (UKPDS 36): prospective observational study. BMJ 2000; 321: 112–119.

29. Gaede P, Vedel P, Parving H-H, Pedersen O. Intensified multifactorial intervention in patients with type 2 diabetes mellitus and microalbuminuria: the Steno type 2 randomised study. Lancet 1999; 353: 617–622.

30. Curb JD, Pressel SL, Cutler JA *et al.* Effect of diuretic-based antihypertensive treatment on cardiovascular risk in older diabetic patients with isolated systolic hypertension. JAMA 1996; 276: 1886–1892.

31. UK Prospective Diabetes Study (UKPDS) Group. Efficacy of atenolol and captopril in reducing risk of macrovascular and microvascular complications in type 2 diabetes: UKPDS 39. BMJ 1998; 317; 713–720.

32. Barzilay JI, Jones CL, Davis BR *et al.* Baseline characteristics of the diabetic participants in the Antihypertensive and Lipid-Lowering Treatment to Prevent Heart Attack trial (ALLHAT). Diabetes Care 2001; 24: 654–658.

33. ALLHAT Officers and Coordinators for the ALLHAT Collaborative Research Group. Major cardiovascular events in hypertensive

patients randomized to doxazosin vs chlorthalidone. JAMA 2000; 283: 1967–1975.

34. Jollis JG, Simpson RJ Jr, Chowdhury MK *et al.* Calcium channel blockers and mortality in elderly patients with myocardial infarction. Arch Intern Med 1999; 159: 2341–2348.

35. Birkenhager WH, Staessen JA. Treatment of diabetic patients with hypertension. Curr Hypertens Rep 1999; 3: 225–231.

36. Tuomilehto J, Rastenyte D, Birkenhager WH *et al.* Effects of calcium-channel blockade in older patients with diabetes and systolic hypertension. N Engl J Med 1999; 340: 677–684.

37. Lindholm LH, Hansson L, Ekbom T *et al.* Comparison of antihypertensive treatments in preventing cardiovascular events in elderly diabetic patients: results from the Swedish Trial in Old Patients with Hypertension – 2. J Hypertens 2000; 18: 1671–1675.

38. Kaplan NM. The management of hypertension in patients with type 2 diabetes. Ann Intern Med 2001; 135: 1079–1083.

39. Tarnow L, Rossing P, Jensen C, Parving H-H. Long-term renoprotective effect of nisoldipine and lisinopril in type 1 diabetic patients with diabetic nephropathy. J Am Soc Nephrol 1999; 10: 134A.

40. Mathiesen ER, Hommel E, Hansen HP *et al.* Randomised controlled trial of long term efficacy of captopril on preservation of kidney function in normotensive patients with insulin dependent diabetes and microalbuminuria. BMJ 1999; 319: 24–25.

41. Hansson L, Lindholm LH, Niskanen L *et al.* Effect of angiotensin-converting-enzyme inhibition compared with conventional therapy on cardiovascular morbidity and mortality in hypertension: the

Captopril Prevention Project (CAPPP) randomised trial. Lancet 1999; 353: 611–616.

42. Gustaffson I, Torp-Pedersen C, Kober L *et al.* for the Trace Study Group. Effect of the angiotensin-converting-enzyme inhibitor trandolapril on mortality and morbidity in diabetic patients with left ventricular dysfunction after acute myocardial infarction. J Am Coll Cardiol 1999; 34: 83–89.

43. Heart Outcomes Prevention Evaluation (HOPE) Study Investigators. Effects of ramipril on cardiovascular and microvascular outcomes in people with diabetes mellitus. Lancet 2000; 355: 253–259.

44. Takai S, Jin D, Sakaguchi M, Miyazaki M. Chymase-dependent angiotensin II formation in human vascular tissue. Circulation 1999; 100: 654–658.

45. Tsutsumi Y, Matsubara H, Masaki H *et al.* Angiotensin II type 2 receptor overexpression activates the vascular kinin system and causes vasodilation. J Clin Invest 1999; 104: 925–935.

46. van Rijnsoever EW, Kwee-Zuiderwijk WJM, Feenstra J. Angioneurotic edema attributed to the use of losartan. Arch Intern Med 1998; 158: 2063–2065.

47. Pitt B, Poole-Wilson PA, Segal R *et al.* Losartan heart failure survival study – ELITE II. Circulation 1999; 100: I-782.

48. Fogari R, Zoppi A, Corradi L *et al.* Adding losartan to lisinopril therapy in patients with hypertension: assessment by 24-hour ambulatory blood pressure monitoring. Curr Therap Res 1999; 60: 326.

49. Mogensen CE, Neldam S, Tikkanen I *et al.* Randomised controlled trial of dual blockade of renin–angiotensin system in patients with hypertension, microalbuminuria, and non-insulin dependent diabetes. BMJ 2000; 321: 1440–1441.

50. Hattori Y, Hattori S, Kasai K. Troglitazone upregulates nitric oxide synthesis in vascular smooth muscle cells. Hypertension 1999; 33: 943–948.

51. Herman WH, Alexander CM, Cook JR et al. Effect of simvastatin treatment on cardiovascular resource utilization in impaired fasting glucose and diabetes. Diabetes Care 1999; 22: 1771–1778.

52. Bakris GK, Williams M, Dworkin L et al. Preserving renal function in adults with hypertension and diabetes. Am J Kidney Dis 2000; 36: 646–661.

7

Arterial compliance: a new measure of therapeutic efficacy

Gary McVeigh, Patrick Allen and David Morgan

Introduction

A number of expert panels have recently published classification schemes and guidelines designed to aid diagnosis, assess severity and determine prognosis in patients with hypertension.[1-3] The recommendations emphasize the role of high blood pressure as a major modifiable cardiovascular risk factor that exhibits a strong, positive and continuous relationship with the risk of cardiovascular disease (stroke, myocardial infarction, heart failure), renal disease and mortality, even within the normotensive range. Clearly, the definition of what constitutes hypertension is arbitrary given the continuous graded relationship between blood pressure and the occurrence of cardiovascular events, but deemed necessary for practical reasons relating to patient assessment and treatment. Whilst the relative risk of cardiovascular events increases with the level of blood pressure, the population attributable risk (a function of relative risk and the percentage of the at-risk population) is greater for lower levels of blood pressure. Thus, the majority of the at-risk population have normal, high-normal or stage 1 hypertension as defined by JNC V1 (*Fig. 7.1*). Given the liability of this measurement in clinical practice, and the minor absolute difference between defined normal and abnormal blood pressure levels, difficulties can arise in deciding who has the disease and in targeting treatment in a cost-effective way to maximize overall cardiovascular risk reduction.

Blood pressure: pulsatile and steady-state components

With the application of the sphygmomanometer to clinical medicine at the beginning of the twentieth century, diastolic blood pressure was initially thought to provide the best measure of cardiovascular risk.[4] Early studies of hypertension approached the arterial circulation as a steady-flow system characterized by mean arterial pressure, which is the product of

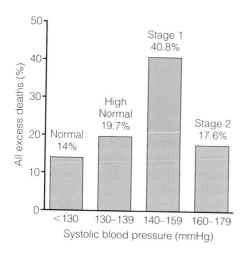

Figure 7.1

Systolic blood pressure and excess all-cause mortality.

cardiac output and total peripheral resistance. Diastolic pressure was taken to mirror peripheral resistance that is viewed as an approximation of the steady-flow load. Increased peripheral resistance has long been regarded as the haemodynamic hallmark of sustained hypertension and has traditionally been employed to monitor the haemodynamic effects of drug interventions.[4] The resistance calculation reflects reduction in capillary density and changes in the wall thickness: lumen ratio of the media of small arteries and arterioles.[5] However, this steady-state haemodynamic approach views the heart as a continuous pump ejecting a constant output into a lumped resistance. Whilst this model describes a stable perfusion pressure and continuous blood flow it ignores the pulsatile component of the haemodynamic load buffered by the compliance characteristics of arterial blood vessels. Recent evidence suggests that the systolic blood pressure and especially the pulse pressure are better predictors of future cardiovascular risk than the diastolic blood pressure.[6] The pulse pressure represents a crude surrogate for alteration in the pulsatile function, or compliance characteristics of the arterial circulation, and is an independent predictor of events for patients with hypertension, congestive cardiac failure or post-myocardial infarction. Thus, the pulsatile function of arteries can no longer be ignored in clinical practice. However, the pulse pressure measurements simply represent the excursions through which pressure fluctuates during the cardiac cycle, and probably reflect established and advanced arterial wall damage. Analysis of the pressure pulse waveform will provide additional information about the interaction of the heart and the arterial circulation, not encompassed in the pulse pressure measurement, that can be detected at an earlier subclinical stage.[7,8]

Experimental studies suggest that the altered vascular architecture described in small arteries may, in large part, be owing to a remodelling process rather than growth.[9] Intuitively, changes in small-artery remodelling and growth would be expected to influence the compliance characteristics of these vessels, in addition to increasing resistance to blood flow. Regarding the large arteries, hypertension can be viewed as an accelerated form of ageing. The pathological changes that occur in the aortic wall, and the associated dilatation and wall thickening, occur at an earlier age if the blood pressure is elevated.[10] Degenerative changes occurring in conduit arteries will not influence the resistance to steady blood flow but will significantly influence the pulsatile pressure load on the heart. Changes in the physical characteristics of large blood vessels will not only alter blood pressure, and especially the pulse pressure, but also cardiac workload, ventricular performance and the arterial pressure pulse contour.[11]

The principle components of blood pressure consist of both a steady component (mean arterial pressure) and a pulsatile component (pulse pressure).[12] The arterial pulse pressure, defined as the difference between the systolic and diastolic blood pressure, is principally a function of stroke volume, arterial compliance and the pattern of ventricular ejection. Pulse pressure at any given ventricular ejection and heart rate will depend on large-artery compliance and the timing and magnitude of peripheral pulse wave reflection. A reduction in arterial compliance or an increase in systemic resistance increases the systolic blood pressure.[13] By contrast, diastolic blood pressure rises with an increase in systemic resistance but falls with impaired compliance characteristics of central arteries; the relative contribution of each parameter determining the ultimate diastolic blood pressure. The fall in diastolic blood pressure associated with a decrease in large-artery compliance is explained by the greater peripheral run-off of the stroke volume during systole and impaired elastic recoil of the aorta to buffer the drop in blood pressure during the diastolic interval.

An understanding of pulsatile and steady state haemodynamic principles is important in order to appreciate the relationship of various blood pressure indices in predicting vascular events and to understand the pathophysiological consequences with respect to the progression of vascular disease. Blood pressure increases progressively with ageing in industrialized societies, beginning in childhood and progressing throughout adulthood.[14] Data from the Framingham Heart Study reveals a concurrent increase in diastolic blood pressure and mean arterial pressure until 50 years of age and a levelling off of diastolic blood pressure between the ages of 50 and 60. After 60 years of age diastolic blood pressure declines (*Fig. 7.2*). Importantly, this change occurs both in normotensive and untreated hypertensive subjects. Systolic blood pressure increases progressively, as does the pulse pressure, with increasing age. Thus, prior to 50 years of age mean arterial pressure, diastolic blood

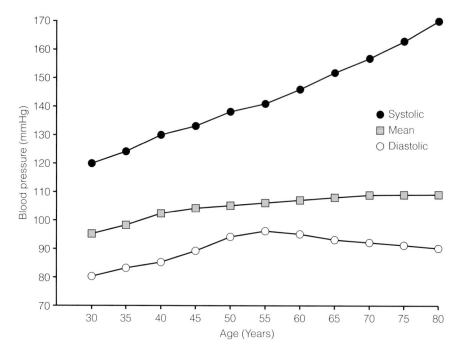

Figure 7.2
Arterial blood pressure components by age

pressure and systolic blood pressure change concordantly. After 50 years of age the relatively greater impairment of arterial compliance leads to a disproportionate increase in systolic blood pressure and pulse pressure, rendering the calculation of mean arterial pressure (two-thirds diastolic blood pressure plus one-third the pulse pressure, in mmHg) inaccurate, leading to an underestimation of total peripheral resistance. An appreciation of pulsatile and steady-state haemodynamics provides a pathophysiological explanation for the paradox of coronary heart disease risk being directly related to diastolic blood pressure when considered alone and inversely related when systolic and diastolic blood pressure are analysed together. These observations suggest that coronary events are most closely related to pulsatile rather than steady stress in the cardiovascular system.

A further consequence of a progressive impairment of large-artery compliance relates to the timing and magnitude of reflected waves in the arterial system. In youth, desirable arterial elastic properties and geometric proportions exist to minimize cardiac work during systole and maintain pressure and flow during diastole, when the heart is not ejecting blood.[15]

The optimal coupling between the left ventricle and the arterial system results in a characteristic pressure pulse contour, where wave reflection from high-impedance-resistance vessels produces a readily apparent secondary pressure rise in late diastole that serves to augment coronary perfusion. With a reduction in large-artery compliance, the forward pressure wave travels with an increased velocity and is reflected from the high-impedance-resistance vessels arriving back at the heart prematurely producing a secondary systolic pressure peak that can augment the systolic blood pressure. This is illustrated graphically in *Fig. 7.3a* and *b*, and it is apparent that the rise in central aortic pressure is disproportionately greater than the rise in peripheral or femoral blood pressure when aortic compliance is reduced. Although the peripheral systolic blood pressure is only 16 mmHg higher in the older subject, central systolic pressure is 30 mmHg higher, while central diastolic pressure is 16 mmHg lower. The pathophysiologic consequence of these changes is a higher left ventricular impedance load and lower coronary perfusion pressure.

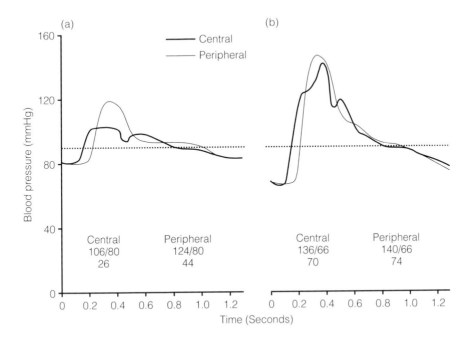

Figure 7.3

Effect of impaired arterial compliance on central and peripheral pulse waveform morphology in (a) young and (b) old subjects.

Arterial compliance and hypertension

Arterial blood vessels are complex three-dimensional structures whose components differ in mechanical, biochemical and physiological characteristics.[16] Arterial wall properties are different in different vessels, differ in the same vessel at various distending pressures and differ with the activation of smooth muscle in the vessel wall. Although no single measure of arterial physical characteristics can completely describe the mechanical behaviour of the vasculature, arterial compliance represents the best clinical index of the buffering function of the arterial system.[17] Arterial compliance is defined as a change in area, diameter or volume for a given change in pressure and is dependent on vessel geometry, in addition to the mechanical properties of the vessel wall. An increase in conduit vessel stiffness significantly influences cardiovascular haemodynamics and alters cardiac workload, ventricular performance, blood pressure and the arterial pressure pulse contour. The abnormalities in pulsatile haemodynamics may also play an important role in the distribution, development and manifestation of atherosclerosis in patients with risk factors known to independently impair arterial compliance characteristics. The possible clinical applications of arterial compliance are outlined in *Fig. 7.4.*

Changes in pulsatile arterial function can influence the growth and remodelling of the left ventricle, large arteries, small arteries and arterioles. Left ventricular mass has been shown to be associated with abnormal pulsatile function independent of body size, age, gender or blood pressure.[18] The origins of small-artery remodelling and the diminished

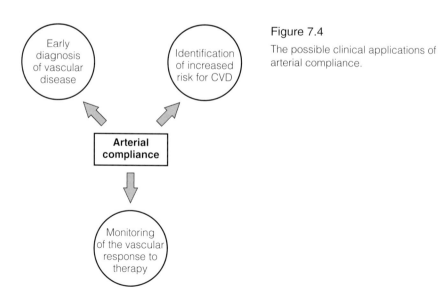

Figure 7.4

The possible clinical applications of arterial compliance.

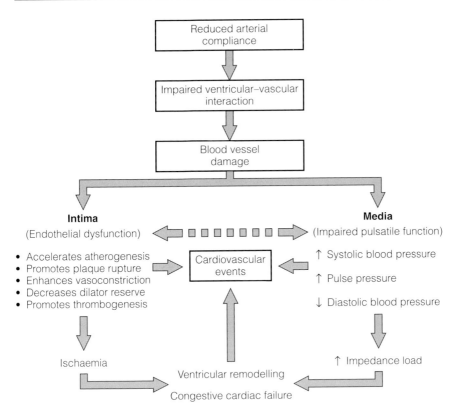

Figure 7.5

Schematic depiction showing the pathophysiological consequences of a reduced arterial compliance.

flow-reserve characteristic of hypertension may reside in the direct effects of high pulsatile stress in these small vessels, or through adverse effects on the endothelium that will influence vascular tone and growth.[19,20] Clearly, arterial blood vessels can no longer be considered as passive conduits to deliver blood to the peripheral tissues in response to metabolic demand. Instead they should be viewed as biophysical sensors that respond to haemodynamic and neurohumoral stimuli that influence the tone and structure of blood vessels. The pathophysiological consequences of impaired compliance characteristics of arterial blood vessels are outlined in *Fig. 7.5*.

Progress in the study of pulsatile arterial function has been hindered by the lack of a gold standard for estimating the buffering function or compliance characteristics of arteries.[17] Each technique employed has inherent limitations and many are invasive and therefore of limited value for clinical studies (*Table 7.1*). Furthermore, conflicting results reported in the medical literature in studies addressing the compliance characteristics of the arterial vasculature with ageing and disease relate to confusion with the usage of terms describing vessel wall mechanical properties, diversity of methods used and heterogeneity of the patient populations and vascular regions studied. These data emphasize the need for validation and development of new non-invasive techniques that are simple to use and provide reproducible measures of pulsatile arterial function that can be applied to the clinical setting to study large numbers of patients in a prospective manner.[6] These technologies should measure aspects of blood vessel pathophysiology and improve the prediction of risk of clinical disease above the traditional measurement of blood pressure. The most promising techniques to date that exhibit feasibility in terms of cost and ease of use involve the measurement of pulse wave velocity and pulse wave analysis.

It is well recognized that a pressure pulse wave is transmitted more slowly in a distensible than in a rigid tube.[21] The measurement of pulse wave velocity refers to estimation of the time of travel of the foot of the pressure, or flow pulse waveform, over a known distance. The foot is defined as the point at the end of diastole when a steep rise of the wave front begins. Mathematical equations are employed to quantitatively express the relationship between pulse wave velocity and elastic modulus, an intrinsic measure of the stiffness of vessel wall constituents.[15] The formulae assume that the pulse wave velocity depends only on vessel diameter, blood density and local arterial wall properties. A change in pulse wave velocity with increased stiffness of arteries does not strictly represent a measure of the compliance characteristics of the arteries, which is defined as an increment in volume produced by an increment in pressure. Furthermore, pulse wave velocity is proportional to the square root of arterial wall stiffness and therefore may not be particularly sensitive to changes in intrinsic wall properties that influence large-vessel compliance. The measurement is also sensitive to changes in heart rate, blood pressure and wave reflection in the arterial system.

There is increasing interest in the descriptive and quantitative analysis of the arterial pulse contour to provide information about generalized changes in the pulsatile characteristics of large and small arterial vessels.[22–24] For many years it has been recognized that qualitatively consistent changes in the arterial pulse contour occur in many cardiovascular disease states, and with physiological and pharmacological interventions. In particular, loss of the oscillatory waveform that distorts the proximal part of the diastolic pressure decay from a pure exponential has been consistently identified as a sensitive marker for altered structure or tone in the vasculature, with ageing and disease states associated with an increase in cardiovascular events.[22–26] This morphological feature arises from wave reflection and a damped resonance occurring in the

Table 7.1 Methods used to estimate arterial compliance

Methods	Advantages	Limitations	Information
Direct			
Angiography	Evaluation of aortic segments	Expensive, invasive	Regional aortic compliance
Magnetic resonance imaging	Non-invasive, not limited by acoustic window, can examine multiple segments	Expensive, remote site of BP measurement	Regional aortic compliance
TTE/TEE	TTE non-invasive, reasonable availability	Expensive, TTE limited by acoustic window, operator-dependent techniques; TEE invasive	Regional aortic compliance
Transcutaneous ET/IVUS techniques	Transcutaneous technique non-invasive; reproducible	Operator dependent, IVUS invasive, remote site of BP measurement with ET	Regional compliance of peripheral arteries
Plethysmographic techniques	Non-invasive, clinical research application	Remote site of BP measurement	Compliance of vascular bed under cuff
Indirect			
Stroke volume/pulse pressure ratio	Non-invasive	Need measure of stroke volume and brachial BP	Total arterial compliance
Pulse wave velocity	Non-invasive, reasonable availability, reproducible	Limited to larger arteries, errors due to wave reflections	Segmental arterial compliance
Fourier analysis of pressure and flow waveforms	Standard technique, reproducible	Expensive, invasive	Total arterial compliance
Pulse contour analysis	Non-invasive, reproducible	Measurement of stroke volume	Total arterial compliance

BP, blood pressure; ET, echo-tracking; IVUS, intravascular ultrasound; TTE, transthoracic echocardiography; TEE, transeophageal echocardiography.

arterial tree, with the major sites of reflected waves originating in the smaller arteries and arterioles.[27]

Loss of the oscillatory diastolic waveform is recognized as an early feature of impaired pulsatile arterial function as it can be found in patients at increased cardiovascular risk without alteration in steady-state haemodynamics.[7,8] A steepening of the diastolic decay is also recognized as a characteristic change in pressure pulse waveform morphology indicative of age- or disease-related reduction in large-artery compliance. These changes in the pressure pulse contour morphology can be analysed by computer-based analysis and quantified to provide information about the capacitive function of conduit arteries, smaller arteries and arterioles that represent the predominant site of reflected waves in the arterial bed.[28] Recent technological advances now permit non-invasive tracking of the arterial waveform by employing an acoustic transducer applanted on the radial artery.[29] In health, optimal coupling between the heart and the peripheral vasculature produces a characteristic waveform that changes in a predictable way with ageing, disease and drug interventions. It would appear intuitively appealing to restore this situation in essential hypertension by prescribing drugs that lower arterial pressure by influencing both pulsatile and steady-state haemodynamics to reproduce the waveform morphology that identifies optimal matching between the heart and the systemic circulation.

Techniques have also been described to determine central aortic pressure waveforms from peripheral arterial waveforms.[30] A feature of the central aortic waveform is a late systolic pressure peak that is assumed to represent reflection from the high-impedance-resistance vasculature. This peak may therefore provide insight into the magnitude of wave reflection and its transit time from the reflecting sites back to the aortic root. Augmentation of the incident pressure pulse wave by reflected waves provides a measure in the incremental increase in arterial pressure attributed to pulse wave reflections. However, this may represent a relatively late change in arterial function, marking the presence of advanced arterial disease as morphological changes in the pulse contour have been well described before significant augmentation of the systolic pressure peak occurs.[31]

A reduction in arterial compliance is a well-accepted finding in hypertension, whatever the site and method of measurement.[32] As high blood pressure itself will induce a decrease in arterial compliance, it remains a matter of debate whether the reduction in compliance represents an alteration of wall properties or is merely a consequence of elevated blood pressure. Currently, considerable controversy exists as to whether abnormalities in arterial compliance in hypertensive patients represents an intrinsic change in the arterial wall or merely a reflection of pressure changes, and whether the changes in compliance are located primarily in the large or small vessels.[33] Several tentative observations suggest that a decrease in arterial compliance in essential hypertension is not solely a mechanical consequence of an elevated blood pressure. In patients with isolated systolic and borderline essential hypertension, the observed decrease in arterial compliance may not be fully accounted for by the marginal increase in mean arterial pressure. In established hypertension, compliance estimates appear reduced to the same extent, regardless of the degree of blood pressure elevation.[15] In addition, different drugs exhibit disparate effects on arterial compliance despite similar reductions in blood pressure. Armentano et al.[34] employed a non-linear mathematical model to represent diameter–pressure relationships in the brachial artery to permit comparison of data in hypertensive and normotensive subjects, under isobaric conditions, from pressure–diameter and pressure–compliance curves in the artery. They concluded that the reduced compliance estimates could not be attributed solely to the stretching effect of elevated blood pressure. These observations suggest that factors in addition to the level of blood pressure, either structural or functional in nature, participate in the mechanisms influencing arterial compliance.

However, a reduced arterial compliance in hypertensive patients has not been a universal finding. With blood pressure controlled as a confounding variable, no difference in forearm arterial compliance between hypertensive and normotensive subjects has been reported in prior studies.[35] In particular, a decreased arterial compliance in muscular conduit arteries may not be a prominent feature of hypertension and observations recorded in peripheral arteries cannot be extrapolated to the more elastic central arteries.[36,37] The lumen diameter of the radial, carotid and femoral arteries are not increased in hypertension. That carotid and femoral wall thickness is increased in hypertensive subjects, despite a normal lumen diameter, provides strong evidence for blood-vessel growth in these subjects. Such changes involving alteration in the proportion and mechanical characteristics of wall components would intuitively be expected to influence arterial compliance estimates. Paradoxically, this may not necessarily occur, as a reduction in the elastic modulus of wall constituents may serve to normalize compliance estimates despite an increase in wall thickness.[38] A decrease in the elastic modulus of wall material has been described in small arteries in experimental hypertension and may serve as a means whereby the vasculature can functionally maintain its elastic mechanical properties, despite the relatively increased wall thickness required by the elevated intravascular pressure. However, the extent to which the altered structure measured under in vitro conditions reflects the in vivo situation remains to be determined. Although speculative, it may be that individuals who do not normalize arterial compliance under isobaric conditions, and consequently expose the vessel to high pulsatile stress, are destined to experience early cardiovascular complications.

Therapeutic trials in hypertension have revealed a dissociation between blood pressure control and the prevention of cardiovascular complications.[39] The association between left ventricular hypertrophy and blood pressure elevation is unexpectedly low, suggesting that left ventricular hypertrophy is not a totally pressure-dependent phenomenon.[33] Regression of left ventricular hypertrophy with treatment is also not necessarily pressure dependent. Recent evidence indicates that how the blood pressure is lowered may be important in restoring normal cardiac and vascular structure and function. In a rat model of hypertension, hydralazine and angiotensin-converting-enzyme (ACE) inhibition lowered mean arterial pressure and peripheral resistance comparably, but only the ACE inhibition significantly reduced left ventricular mass.[40] The differential regression of left ventricular hypertrophy was attributed to favourable effects on pulsatile load exhibited solely by the ACE inhibitor. Thus, unrecognized effects on pulsatile haemodynamics may account for the differential effects of various agents on cardiovascular remodelling. Pulse pressure, a correlate of large-vessel compliance, is recognized as an important independent predictor of clinical events in hypertensive patients and in the general population.[6,11,12] The impaired compliance characteristics of arterial blood vessels may promote the development and progression of atherosclerosis, and the effects of continued pulsatile stress on atheromatous plaques may favour rupture and the occurrence of clinical events. Thus, it has been suggested that effective antihypertensive treatment requires normalization of pulsatile and steady-state components of blood pressure to maximize benefits in terms of reversing abnormalities in cardiovascular structure and function in patients with hypertension.[33]

The therapeutic benefits of antihypertensive drugs on arteries consists of two major effects: the effect due to blood pressure lowering and the direct effect of the drug on the vessel wall.[41] Arterial compliance will decrease as blood pressure increases due to the non-linear distensible characteristics of arteries. Unfortunately, most studies cannot differentiate a compliance change attributable to the drug effect on the blood pressure from the direct effect of the drug on the vessel wall. High blood pressure frequently coexists with other cardiovascular risk factors that can increase the risk of vascular events by up to 10-fold.[1–3] These cardiovascular risk factors may independently influence the compliance characteristics of the arterial circulation by altering the structure and function of arterial blood vessels.[42] Drug therapy that favourably influences blood vessel function directly may improve the mechanical properties of the arterial vasculature independent of changes in the blood pressure.

Although the determinants of arterial compliance are incompletely understood, an attractive hypothesis is that altered endothelial function impacts the compliance characteristics of arteries and that pharmacological modulation of endothelial function may improve arterial compliance and perhaps favourably influence clinical outcome. Factors known to

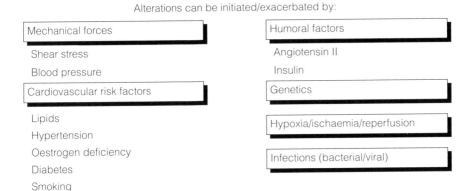

Figure 7.6

The causes of vascular wall remodelling which act primarily by alterations in endothelial function.

influence arterial wall structure and growth, capable of acting primarily through modulating endothelial function, are outlined in *Fig. 7.6*.

The vascular endothelium elaborates relaxing and constricting factors, and growth promoting and inhibiting factors, that profoundly influence structure and tone in the arterial circulation.[43] An imbalance that favours vasoconstriction and vascular growth in blood vessels is found in patients with risk factors for and disease states associated with an increase in cardiovascular events. In particular, impaired nitric oxide-mediated vasodilation has been consistently identified in patients at increased risk for cardiovascular disease.[44] As endothelium-derived nitric oxide is viewed as vasculoprotective, restoration of nitric oxide synthesis and activity is increasingly regarded as a therapeutic target for pharmacological interventions. Impaired pulsatile function of arteries and defective nitric oxide-mediated control of arterial tone are common accompaniments in disease states associated with an increase in cardiovascular events.[24] It has previously been shown that the short-term administration of fish-oil supplements in patients with diabetes mellitus enhances nitric oxide production or activity from the endothelium and significantly improves pulsatile arterial function without influencing cardiac output, total peripheral resistance or blood pressure.[45,46] These data provide support for the concept that therapies which favourably influence endothelial function can improve the pulsatile characteristics of the arterial circulation; a relatively unexplored target that may contribute to the cardiovascular protective actions of drug interventions. Furthermore, it is apparent that vascular adaptations associated with endothelial dysfunction may not be detected by monitoring traditional steady-state haemodynamic variables such as peripheral vascular resistance.

The effects of drug therapy on arterial compliance are complex and involve a number of competing mechanisms. Therefore, it is not surprising that studies of arterial compliance in different species, different arteries or different disease states have produced conflicting results. The technical and methodological limitations in the largely cross-sectional studies that have evaluated changes in arterial compliance with drug therapy should therefore be interpreted only in a general and directional way. Glasser et al.[41] (Table 7.2) have recently reviewed the effects of individual drugs and classes of drugs on the compliance characteristics of arteries in patients with hypertension.[41] Analysis of these studies clearly indicates that arterial compliance in hypertension is modifiable and that alteration in the compliance characteristics of arteries is not exclusively dependent on a decrease in blood pressure with therapy. ACE inhibition in hypertensive patients decreases blood pressure and wave reflection, and improves arterial compliance.[47] Low-dose diuretics can also be effective agents in improving the compliance characteristics of arteries, to an extent similar to that seen with ACE inhibitors.[48] Nitrovasodilators uniformly improve the compliance characteristics of arteries, in contrast to direct-acting vasodilators (e.g. hydralazine) which do not increase arterial compliance despite decreasing blood pressure.[41] Calcium antagonists, in the short-term at least, appear to benefit wave reflection and arterial compliance, although the long-term benefits are the subject of debate.[49] Overall, β-receptor antagonists appear to have little beneficial effect on arterial compliance in short- or longer term studies.[50] These latter observations concerning the modest effects of β-blockade in favourably influencing arterial pulsatile function have to be weighed against the proven benefits of these compounds in large-scale clinical outcome studies. Certainly, drug therapy that lowers the blood pressure in hypertensive patients would be expected to improve clinical outcome. Whether further improvements in outcome depend on how the blood pressure is lowered (by influencing both pulsatile and steady-state haemodynamics) or by favourably influencing the arterial wall (through direct effects on the endothelium) requires further study. What is now required are large-scale prospective outcome studies that relate abnormal compliance and direct vascular effects of drug interventions to clinical outcome in patients with essential hypertension.

Hypertension should be viewed primarily as a vascular disease characterized by structural and functional changes in the cardiovascular system. At present, diagnostic procedures are designed to assess the extent and severity of blood vessel damage when symptoms present, or with the occurrence of vascular events. Traditional cuff sphygmomanometry describes the excursions through which pressure fluctuates during the cardiac cycle but it is not a sensitive guide to the extent of end-organ damage due to degeneration or disease in arterial walls. Even the fortuitous detection of target-organ damage by clinical examination, mani-

Table 7.2 Antihypertensive drug-class effects on arterial compliance in humans

Drug class	No. of agents tested	No. of studies*	No. of patients	Increase in arterial compliance yielded
Calcium channel blockers (CCB)	8	11	~150	With all agents
β-Blockers	7	10	~326	None, except 'vasodilating' β-blockers
ACE inhibitors	8	14	~260	With all agents studied (most were perindopril)
Diuretics	4	5	~75	Little effect beyond that associated with decreasing BP (an attempt was made methodologically to separate pressure-dependent from direct effects)
Nitrovasodilators	2	2	27	Some effect
Direct vasodilators	3	3	Review	With none
α-Blockers	1	1	12	Some effect
Clonidine	1	1	12	No effect
Oestrogen	1	1	78	Some effect

*Studies are primarily cross-sectional and short term. Thus, these studies can only be used for information regarding directional effects and, by and large, cannot distinguish functional from structural changes. BP, blood pressure.
(Modified from Glasser et al.[41])

fested by changes in retinal blood vessels, the presence of arterial bruits or detection of left ventricular hypertrophy, represents an advanced stage in the disease process. The diagnostic challenge must be to detect abnormal structure and function in the vascular system at an early pre-clinical stage. New diagnostic techniques facilitate the identification of early pathophysiological changes in arteries that may predate, or be associated with, an elevated blood pressure but not identified by cuff sphygmomanometry. The ability to detect and monitor subclinical arterial damage has the potential to improve cardiovascular risk stratification and act as a better guide in assessing the efficacy of therapeutic interventions than monitoring blood pressure alone.

References

1. The sixth report of the Joint National Committee on Prevention, Detection, Evaluation and treatment of high blood pressure. Arch Intern Med 1997; 157: 2413–2446.

2. World Health Organization – International Society of Hypertension (WHO-ISH). WHO-ISH Guidelines for the Management of Hypertension. J Hypertens 1999; 17: 151–183

3. Ramsey LE, Williams B, Johnston GD et al. Guidelines for management of hypertension: report of the third working party of the British Hypertension Society. J Hum Hypertens 1999; 13: 569–592.

4. MacWilliams JA. Systolic and diastolic blood pressure estimation. BMJ 1914; 2: 693–697.

5. Folkow B. The fourth Volhard lecture. Cardiovascular structural adaptation: its role in initiation and maintenance of primary hypertension. Clin Sci Molec Med 1978; 55 (suppl 2): 2S–22S.

6. Black HR, Kuller LH, O'Rourke MF et al. The first report of the Systolic and Pulse Pressure (SYPP) Working Group. J Hypertens 1999; 17 (suppl 5): S3–S14.

7. McVeigh G, Brennan G, Hayes R et al. Vascular abnormalities in non-insulin-dependent diabetes mellitus identified by arterial waveform analysis. Am J Med 1993; 95: 424–430.

8. McVeigh GE, Morgan DJ, Finkelstein SM et al. Vascular abnormalities associated with long-term cigarette smoking identified by arterial waveform analysis. Am J Med 1997; 102: 227–231.

9. Baumbach GL, Heistad DD. Remodeling of cerebral arterioles in chronic hypertension. Hypertension 1989; 13: 968–972.

10. Wolinsky H. Long-term effects of hypertension on rat aortic wall and their relation to concurrent aging changes: morphological and chemical studies. Circ Res 1972; 30: 301–309.

11. Mitchell GF, Pfeffer MA. Pulsatile hemodynamics in hypertension. Curr Opin Cardiol 1999; 14: 361–369.

12. Franklin SS, Khan SA, Wong ND et al. Is pulse pressure useful in predicting risk for coronary heart disease? The Framingham Heart Study. Circulation 1999; 100: 354–360.

13. Nichols WW, Nicoline FA, Pepine CJ. Determinants of isolated systolic hypertension in the elderly. J

Hypertens 1992; 10 (suppl 6): 573–577.

14. Franklin SS, Gustin WG, Wong ND et al. Hemodynamic patterns of age-related changes in blood pressure. The Framingham Heart Study. Circulation 1997; 96: 308–315.

15. McVeigh GE, Bank AJ, Cohn JN. Vascular compliance. In: Willerson JT, Cohn JN, eds. Cardiovascular medicine. Churchill Livingstone: Philadelphia, 1995, 1212–1227.

16. Lee RT, Kamm RD. Vascular mechanics for the cardiologist. J Am Coll Cardiol 1994; 23: 1289–1295.

17. McVeigh GE. Evaluation of arterial compliance. In: Izzo JL Jr, Black HR, eds. Hypertension primer, 2nd edn. American Heart Association: Dallas, 1999, 327–329.

18. Saba PS, Roman MJ, Pini R et al. Relation of arterial pressure waveform to left ventricular and carotid anatomy in normotensive subjects. J Am Coll Cardiol 1993; 22: 1873–1880.

19. Ryan SM, Waack BJ, Weno BL, Heistad DD. Increases in pulse pressure impair acetylcholine-induced vascular relaxation. Am J Physiol 1995; 268: H359–H363.

20. Cheng GC, Loree HM, Kamm RD et al. Distribution of circumferential stress in ruptured and stable atherosclerotic lesions: a structural analysis with histopathological correlation. Circulation 1993; 87: 1179–1187.

21. Bramwell JC, Hill AV. Velocity of transmission of the pulse wave and elasticity of arteries. Lancet 1922; 1: 891–892.

22. Fries ED, Heath WC, Luchsinger PC, Snell RE. Changes in the carotid pulse which occur with age and hypertension. Am Heart J 1966; 71: 757–765.

23. Kelly R, Hayward C, Avolio A, O'Rourke M. Noninvasive determination of age-related changes in the human arterial pulse. Circulation 1989; 80: 1652–1659.

24. McVeigh GE, Bratteli CW, Morgan DJ et al. Age-related abnormalities in arterial compliance identified by pressure pulse contour analysis. Aging and arterial compliance. Hypertension 1999; 33: 1392–1398.

25. Cohn JN, Finkelstein S, McVeigh G et al. Noninvasive pulse wave analysis for the early detection of vascular disease. Hypertension 1995; 26: 503–508.

26. Lax H, Feinburg AW. Abnormalities of the arterial pulse wave in young diabetic subjects. Circulation 1959; 20: 1106–1110.

27. Nichols WW, O'Rourke MF. Contours of pressure and flow waves in arteries. In: Nichols WW, O'Rourke MF, eds. McDonalds blood flow in arteries, 4th edn. Oxford University Press: New York, 1998, 170–201.

28. Watt TB, Burrus CS. Arterial pressure contour analysis for estimating human vascular properties. J Appl Physiol 1976; 40: 171–176.

29. Cohn JN. Vascular wall function as a risk marker for cardiovascular disease. J Hypertens 1999; 17 (suppl 5): S41–S44.

30. Nichols WW, O'Rourke MF. Sphygmocardiography. In: Nichols WW, O'Rourke MF, eds. McDonalds blood flow in arteries, 4th edn. Oxford University Press: New York, 1998, 450–476.

31. Murgo JP, Westerhof N, Giolima JT, Altobelli SA. Aortic input impedance in normal man: relationship to pressure waveforms. Circulation 1980; 62: 105–116.

32. Simon A, Levenson J. Use of arterial compliance for evaluation of hypertension. Am J Hypertens 1991; 4: 97–105.

33. Glasser SP, Arnett DK, McVeigh GE et al. Vascular compliance

and cardiovascular disease. A risk factor or a marker. Am J Hypertens 1997; 10: 1175–1189.

34. Armentano R, Simon A, Levenson J et al. Mechanical pressure versus intrinsic effects of hypertension on large arteries in humans. Hypertension 1991; 18: 657–666.

35. Gribben B, Pickering TG, Sleight P. Arterial distensibility in normal and hypertensive man. Clin Sci 1979; 56: 413–417.

36. Weber R, Sterglopulos N, Brunner HR, Hayoz D. Contributions of vascular tone and structure to elastic properties of a medium-sized artery. Hypertension 1996; 27: 816–822.

37. Khder Y, Bray Des Boscs L, Aliot E, Zannad F. Endothelial, viscoelastic and sympathetic factors contributing to arterial wall changes during aging. Cardiol Elderly 1996; 4: 161–165.

38. Mulvany MJ. A reduced elastic modulus of vascular wall components in hypertension? Hypertension 1992; 20: 7–9.

39. McVeigh GE, Burns DE, Finkelstein SM et al. Reduced vascular compliance as a marker for essential hypertension. Am J Hypertens 1991; 4: 245–251.

40. Mitchell GF, Pfeffer MA, Finn PV, Pfeffer JM. Equipotent antihypertensive agents variously affect pulsatile hemodynamics and regression of cardiac hypertrophy in spontaneously hypertensive rats. Circulation 1996; 94: 2923–2929.

41. Glasser SP, Arnett DK, McVeigh GE et al. The importance of arterial compliance in cardiovascular drug therapy. J Clin Pharmacol 1998; 38: 202–212.

42. Nutel JM, Smith DH, Grattinger WF, Weber MA. Dependency of arterial compliance on circulating neuroendocrine and metabolic factors in normal subjects. Am J Cardiol 1992; 69: 1340–1344.

43. De Meyer GRY, Herman AG. Vascular endothelial dysfunction. Prog Cardiovasc Dis 1997; 34: 325–342.

44. Luscher TF, Noll G. Endothelial function as an end-point in international trials: concepts, methods and current data. J Hypertens 1996; 145 (suppl 2): S111–S121.

45. McVeigh GE, Brennan GM, Johnston GD et al. Dietary fish oil augments nitric oxide production or release in patients with Type 2 (non-insulin-dependent) diabetes mellitus. Diabetologia 1993; 36: 33–38.

46. McVeigh GE, Brennan GM, Cohn JN et al. Fish oil improves arterial compliance in non-insulin dependent diabetes mellitus. Arterioscler Thromb 1994; 14: 1425–1429.

47. Safar ME, van Bortel LM, Struijker-Boudier HA. Resistance and conduit arteries following converting enzyme inhibition in hypertension. J Vasc Res 1997; 34: 67–81.

48. Girerd X, Giannattasio C, Moulin C et al. Regression of radial artery wall hypertrophy and improvement of carotid artery wall compliance after long-term antihypertensive treatment in elderly patients. J Am Coll Cardiol 1998; 31: 1064–1073.

49. De Cesaris R, Ranieri G, Filitti V, Andriani A. Large artery compliance in essential hypertension: effects of calcium antagonism and beta-blocking. Am J Hypertens 1992; 5: 624–628.

50. Pannier BM, Lafleche AB, Girerd XJM et al. Arterial stiffness and wave reflections following acute calcium blockade in essential hypertension. Am J Hypertens 1994; 7: 168–176.

8

Treatment of hypertension to prevent atherosclerosis

Chiara Bolego, Andrea Poli and Rodolfo Paoletti

Introduction

Hypertension, a primary risk factor for the development of atherosclerosis,[1] is not only a disease of blood pressure but rather is a progressive process of structural changes in the vasculature with alterations in the endothelial functions. Therefore, lowering blood pressure is not the sole therapeutic target in patients with hypertension. In particular, attention should be directed to drugs with multiple effects, which share both blood-pressure-lowering properties and vascular protection.

Since endothelial damage plays a key role in the development of hypertension as well as atherosclerosis,[2] drugs affecting endothelial functions should be effective in reducing clinical events such as myocardial infarction (MI), stroke and peripheral vascular disease. In this chapter vascular protective properties will be discussed, both antihypertensive and antiatherosclerotic properties of different classes of drugs such as calcium-channel blockers (CCB), angiotensin-converting-enzyme (ACE) inhibitors, sartanes, third-generation β-blockers and statins. The outstanding clinical trials in this field will also be reviewed. Event-based trials of antihypertensive therapy, although essential in showing the beneficial effects of antihypertensive therapy on cardiovascular morbidity and mortality, are unable to answer the question of whether antihypertensive therapy influences the development of atherosclerosis. Trials based on event and end-organ damage, using measurements of plaque growth as end-points, are of particular interest. Moreover, on the basis of the mechanisms of action of these classes of drugs, the clinical relevance of combined treatment will be also taken into account.

Endothelial function in hypertension and atherosclerosis

Vascular endothelial cells play a key role in the regulation of cardiovascular function by producing a number of potent vasodilator molecules, e.g.

129

nitric oxide (NO) and prostacyclin (PGI_2), and vasoconstrictor agents, e.g. endothelin (ET-1), thromboxane A_2 (TXA_2) and angiotensin II (Ang II), both of which contribute to the maintenance of physiological vascular tone. A dysfunction of the vascular endothelium has been implicated in the pathophysiology of a number of cardiovascular diseases such as hypertension. Hypercholesterolemia and diabetes may also be associated with reduced endothelial function in the absence of elevated blood pressure. All these pathological conditions, which start from an endothelial impairment, represent important risk factors for atherosclerosis and an increased risk of cardiovascular events.

Indeed, atherosclerosis develops as a later manifestation of endothelial dysfunction and its progression is influenced by many risk factors which are often present in individuals with hypertension.

Modulation of endothelial function is therefore an important therapeutic option in the treatment of hypertension to prevent atherosclerosis and clinical events, such as myocardial infarction (MI), stroke and claudicatio intermittens.

NO is secreted from the endothelium after the stimulation of the constitutive form of nitric oxide synthase (cNOS), in response to different physiological and pharmacological stimuli such as acetylcholine, bradykinin and exercise, and its production contributes to physiological vasodilation. However, in patients with hypertension who are prone to develop cardiovascular events, an impairment of NO-mediated endothelium-dependent relaxation occurs. This is mainly due to reduced NO secretion from the endothelium but may also result from increased inactivation of NO by superoxide radicals. Otherwise, NO may be secreted from smooth muscle cells after stimulation of the inducible form of NO synthase (iNOS) in response to pro-inflammatory stimuli such as cytokines and interferon (IFN)-γ. Induction of iNOS produces a high output of NO, which is transformed into toxic metabolites such as peroxynitrite (superoxide anions). Reduced production of NO by endothelium and increased iNOS activation, which leads to an excessive production of free radicals, have been implicated in the development of atherosclerosis.[3]

A functional feedback balance exists between Ang II and NO under normal conditions. The NO–Ang II imbalance alone may not explain the vascular pathophysiology of hypertension but it certainly appears to be an important component. The endothelial response to hypotension is to organize a complex local environment, including upregulation of NO and inhibition of the effects of Ang II, in order to preserve end-organ damage.

Endothelial cells contain Ang II-converting-enzyme (ACE), which convert Ang I to Ang II, a potent vasoconstrictor with growth-promoting properties. NO is a potent vasodilator with antigrowth and antithrombogenic properties and has been shown to downregulate the synthesis of ACE in the endothelium,[4] as well as Ang II-type receptors (AT_1) in the smooth muscle cells,[5] thus having the potential to decrease Ang II production and action. ACE inhibitors not only decrease Ang II synthesis, but also prevent the degradation of bradykinin, one of the most important molecules involved in the release of NO.

The development and/or maintenance of both hypertension and the abnormal vascular remodeling that occurs in atherosclerosis and after myocardial injury is probably due, in part, to the loss of NO and, more importantly, to an imbalance of Ang II, NO and superoxide anion production.[6] The reasons for the imbalance between these substances are often unclear. An understanding of the relationships between hypertension, end-organ damage and the Ang II–NO axis leads to the belief that currently available therapeutic strategies capable of restoring the homeostatic balance of these vasoactive agents within the vessel wall would be effective in preventing or arresting end-organ disease.

The absence of clinically applicable methodology to evaluate the state of the arterial vasculature has inhibited the development of markers, other than blood pressure, for the diagnosis and treatment of hypertension. At present, the direct visualization of arteries using new ultrasound techniques has provided the opportunity to measure the intimal–medial thickness and to assess the compliance of visualized blood vessels.[7] An increased media/lumen ratio indeed represents an important feature of the vascular remodeling, a dynamic process of adaptation of the vascular beds to both hypertension and atherosclerosis.

The evaluation of structural alterations in the arteries provides a useful guide to the risk of cardiovascular events and underlines the importance of antihypertensive therapies directed to preserve the progressive structural abnormalities of the vascular wall.

Antihypertensive drugs with additional effects on the arterial wall

Hypertension involves three major factors: abnormal vascular tone, abnormalities in volume and salt regulation, and vessel wall remodeling. Both NO and Ang II are important players in the vascular remodeling process, which relates directly to cardiovascular morbidity and mortality. Drugs like Ang II inhibitors, Ang-receptor (AT_1) blockers (ARB), calcium antagonists, β-blockers and statins, which directly regulate or interfere with the regulation of these molecules, will be able to act as antihypertensives not only by reducing blood pressure but, more importantly, by acting on the arterial wall and so preventing end-organ damage related to hypertension. Several of these drugs also share other important mechanisms of action, such as cell-growth-inhibiting properties or reduction of molecules (ET-1), which enhance vascular tone and further contribute to oppose vascular wall abnormalities. These effects have frequently been described as pleiotropic actions.

ACE inhibitors

ACE inhibitors (ACEI) are a class of drugs that have favourable vasopro-tective properties which not only depend on the hypotensive effect related to the inhibition of Ang II production and the increased bioavail-ability of bradykinin. Indeed, ACEI have been shown to reduce the risk of coronary events in various patient groups and to prevent the develop-ment of atherosclerosis in animal models.

ACE regulates the balance between the renin–angiotensin system (RAS) and the kallikrein system. In the case of cardiovascular artery dis-ease (CAD), hypertension and cardiovascular heart failure (CHF), activa-tion of the RAS causes long-term activation of Ang and degradation of bradykinin, resulting in secondary, permanent structural changes that are peculiar to these chronic pathological conditions.[6]

Several mechanisms could be responsible for these effects. ACE inhi-bition prevents stimulation of Ang II receptors on smooth muscle cells, thus blocking both smooth muscle cell contraction and proliferation. Moreover, as a consequence of a reduced bradykinin breakdown and the activation of bradykinin type 2 receptors, ACEI enhance NO and PGI_2 production. ACE inhibition also diminishes the production of superoxide anions, which inactivate NO, further contributing to enhanced NO bioavailability. An inhibitory effect of ACEI on endothelin-1 has also been described, further supporting a cardioprotective role for these drugs.[8] Thus, ACEI promote vasodilatory, antithrombotic and antiproliferative effects, leading to a general protection against atherosclerosis develop-ment.

In patients with CAD, ramipril and losartan improve endothelial function by enhancing NO bioavailability due to an increased activity of superox-ide dismutase (SOD), the major antioxidant enzyme of the arterial wall.[9] Despite these effects and the well-documented reduction of cardiovascu-lar mortality in patients with MI and CHF,[10] at present few clinical data demonstrate a reduction on carotid or coronary atherosclerosis after ACEI treatment. The HOPE study evaluated the effects of ramipril in patients with established atherosclerotic disease and showed a reduction of fatal and non-fatal events, unrelated to blood pressure reduction.[11] The SECURE trial, a substudy of the HOPE trial, recently demonstrated that long-term treatment with ramipril had a beneficial effect on atherosclero-sis progression.[12] In contrast, the SCAT study failed to demonstrate any angiographic effect of enalapril on coronary atherosclerosis in normocho-lesterolemic patients.[13] Similarly, in patients with coronary, cerebrovascu-lar or peripheral disease treated with ramipril, no changes in carotid atherosclerosis were observed.[14]

The Plaque Hypertension Lipid Lowering Italian Study (PHYLLIS) is the first study in patients with hypertension, moderate hypercholesterolemia and initial carotid artery alterations which investigates whether, in these patients, the combined administration of an ACEI (fosinopril) and a statin (pravastatin) is more effective than the administration of a diuretic and a lipid-lowering diet in retarding or regressing the alterations in carotid IMT. This study is still in progress but baseline data clearly indicate an association between blood pressure elevation and carotid artery alterations in this population.[15]

AT$_1$ receptor antagonists (sartanes)

Ang II binds at least two specific receptors: Ang II type 1 and 2 receptors (AT$_1$ and AT$_2$). AT$_1$ mediates the vasoconstrictor effect of Ang II and the Ang II-induced growth in cardiovascular tissue.[16] Sartanes represent a new class of antihypertensive drugs that selectively block the AT$_1$ receptor and, similarly to ACEI, are thought to possess pleiotropic effects responsible for end-organ protection. Insulin is elevated in non-insulin-dependent diabetes mellitus (NIDDM) and in patients with plurimetabolic syndrome. Insulin stimulates the upregulation of vascular AT$_1$ receptor gene expression, thus sensitizing the arterial wall to the action of Ang II, as reflected by the frequent association between glucose tolerance, hypertension and atherosclerosis.[6] Sartanes may therefore be interesting for the control of high blood pressure in patients at higher cardiovascular risk.

Different pleiotropic effects of sartanes have been described in experimental models. For instance, candesartan at low doses has been shown to normalize NOS production and to improve the vascular morphology in hypertensive rats.[17] In addition, sartanes suppress AT$_1$-dependent oxidative bursts of macrophages, which may contribute to their antiatherosclerotic effects. It is worthwhile mentioning that by blocking AT$_1$ receptors, sartanes leave the AT$_2$ receptor effects unopposed. For instance, AT$_2$ receptors activate several tyrosine phosphatases and serine/threonine phosphatases, thus suppressing cell growth mechanisms.[16]

So far, however, there are no clinical data demonstrating that sartanes reduce the morbidity and mortality associated with the clinical manifestations of atherosclerosis.

Calcium-channel blockers (CCB)

Calcium antagonists are frequently used in the treatment of hypertension and also have an antiatherogenic potential unrelated to their calcium-channel blocking properties, which have been demonstrated in various experimental models. Lacidipine, a third-generation lipophilic calcium antagonist, may directly interfere with major processes of atherogenesis occurring in the arterial wall.[18] Nifedipine increases endothelium-dependent vasodilation by enhancing NO availability, probably due to its antioxidant activity.[19]

However, there are conflicting clinical data on the beneficial effects of antihypertensive CCB on the progression of atherosclerosis, as well as on the reduction of clinical events.[20]

The PREVENT trial was not able to demonstrate any effect of amlodipine on angiographic progression of atherosclerosis or the risk of major cardiovascular events.[21] However, it would appear that quantitative angiography may not be appropriate for monitoring the progression of atherosclerosis, due to arterial remodeling processes. The VHAS study demonstrated that verapamil is more effective than the diuretic clortalidone in promoting the regression of thicker carotid lesions.[22] The European Lacidipine Study of Atherosclerosis (ELSA) is a multinational interventional trial in progress to determine the effect of 4 years of treatment with the calcium antagonist lacidipine versus the β-blocker atenolol on the progression of carotid atherosclerosis in asymptomatic patients. There is a marked prevalence of carotid artery atherosclerosis in asymptomatic patients. There is a marked prevalence of carotid artery wall alterations among mild to moderate middle-aged hypertensive patients.[23] Results of ELSA (presented at the European Congress of Hypertension)[15] clearly indicate a similar reduction of blood pressure in patients treated with lacidipine and atenolol, but only lacidipine inhibits the increased thickness of the carotid vessels.

Third-generation β-blockers

Carvedilol and nebivolol are multiple-action cardiovascular drugs that are currently used in many countries for the treatment of hypertension. Besides its β-adrenergic blocking and vasodilating properties, carvedilol, and even more so its metabolites, is a potent antioxidant. This activity may account for the cardioprotective effects of carvedilol in pathological conditions such as hypertension and coronary artery disease, in which oxidative stress is recognized to occur. It has been demonstrated that long-term treatment with carvedilol improves endothelium-dependent vasodilation in brachial arteries, probably due to its antioxidant potential.[24]

Nebivolol is a highly selective and lipophilic β_1 receptor antagonist with vasodilating characteristics which has recently been demonstrated to inhibit the proliferation of endothelial cells and to enhance NO synthesis.[25] Both carvedilol and nebivolol have been shown also to inhibit proliferation of human coronary smooth muscle cells and ET-1 release in a concentration-dependent manner.[26] *In vivo*, metabolized nebivolol increases vascular NO production.[27] Therefore, these antihypertensive drugs show several characteristics of a modern pharmacological agent to treat cardiovascular disease, preserving the endothelial integrity, inhibiting cell growth and blocking the oxidative burst.

The CAPRICORN study, a multicentre randomized trial, demonstrated that the addition of carvedilol to standard therapies for the treatment of acute MI in patients with left ventricular dysfunction, with or without heart failure, would improve outcome in terms of mortality and morbidity,[28] supporting the idea that carvedilol provides a mechanism to further reduce mortality in high-risk patients.

Statins

High serum cholesterol has frequently been reported in patients with arterial hypertension, leading to an exponential increase in cardiovascular risk. Several clinical trials have demonstrated that the competitive inhibitors of HMG-CoA reductase (statins) reduce cardiovascular mortality.

Independent of their lipid-lowering properties, statins are known to have several important direct vascular effects, which may have an impact on cardiovascular pathophysiology. Several properties are common to all statins, while, at least *in vitro*, others seem to be molecule specific. Even though there are concerns about the pleiotropic effects of HMG-CoA inhibitors, and several investigators relate all of these actions to the reduction of plasma cholesterol levels, *in vitro* studies clearly show a direct vascular effects of statins.

For instance, atorvastatin and simvastatin improve endothelial function *in vitro* independently from their lipid-lowering effect, as demonstrated by the upregulation of endothelial NOS (eNOS).[29] Indeed, the enhanced eNOS activity by statins is the predominant mechanism by which these agents protect against cerebral injury, as demonstrated by the loss of the effect in eNOS-deficient mice.[30] Fluvastatin reduces the secretion of endothelin in human vein endothelial cells in culture, further supporting a direct favourable role of these class of drugs on the vascular wall.[31]

Moreover, it has been shown that statins inhibit endothelial O_2^- formation, enhancing NO formation and improving endothelial function.[32] The augmented bioactivity of NO by statins might account not only for enhancement of endothelium-dependent vasodilation but also for other antiatherogenic effects of statins, such as the inhibition of platelet aggregation and the release of factors that stimulate growth and migration of smooth muscle cells within the vessel wall.[33] With the exception of the hydrophilic pravastatin, smooth muscle cell proliferation in culture is negatively regulated by sera of patients treated with statins.[34] Interestingly, fluvastatin reduces ACE activity in cholesterol-fed rabbits; this effect further contributes to a decreased risk in atherosclerosis progression.[35]

The comparison of experimental and clinical data for this class of drugs suggest that the activities of single statins studied *in vitro* cannot be extrapolated to the clinical situation. Indeed, clinical trials fail to show direct vascular effects. However, the AFCAPS/TexCAPS study confirms that additional mechanisms, other than lipid lowering, play a relevant part in the action of statins.[36]

In clinical studies using HMG-CoA reductase inhibitors, improved vasodilating properties of the vessels were reported. Recently, it has been published that statins in combination with other antihypertensive drugs can improve blood pressure control in patients with uncontrolled hypertension and high serum cholesterol levels. The authors suggest that the additional blood pressure reduction observed in treated patients is only partially related to statins' lipid-lowering effects.[37] Moreover, a study by Tonolo et al.[38] shows that simvastatin but not cholestyramine therapy in hypertensive type 2 diabetic patients was able to reduce blood pressure, suggesting a mechanism independent from low-density lipoprotein (LDL) cholesterol reduction. In hypercholesterolemic postmenopausal women treated with atorvastatin a significant improvement in endothelial reactivity has been demonstrated, but the extent to which this was related to cholesterol reduction or to a direct effect remains to be established.[39] Moreover, Nazzaro et al.[40] demonstrated that enalapril and simvastatin, when given together to hypertensive and hypercholesterolemic patients, have additive effects on vascular reactivity and structural damage. Finally, in hypercholesterolemic patients on treatment with enalapril or lisinopril an additional fall in blood pressure was observed when lovastatin or pravastatin was added to the therapy.[41]

The emerging wide range of properties related to statins provide the basis for explaining benefits beyond those observed with cholesterol lowering. These activities contribute to the maintenance of the endothelium integrity, affecting both vasodilation and the formation of atherosclerotic lesions. In particular, HMG-CoA reductase inhibitors could represent an additional tool for the treatment of normocholesterolemic patients with hypertension.

Future clinical trials designed to evaluate the pleiotropic effects of statins will definitively clarify the relative contribution of the direct vascular effects of statins to clinical outcome.

Conclusions

Decisions about the management of hypertensive patients should not be based on blood pressure alone but also on the presence of other risk factors, target-organ damage and cardiovascular disease. In this perspective, non-invasive ultrasound examination of patients could add important information about their pathological conditions; clinical studies designed for the evaluation of vascular wall alterations with angiographic techniques could better define the efficacy of several classes of drugs.

It is clear that several classes of antihypertensive drugs have additional mechanisms which may counteract the development of atherosclerosis, therefore reducing cardiovascular morbidity and mortality.

Moreover, statins, beyond their lipid-lowering properties, are known to have pleiotropic effects which contribute to their vascular protective profile. A growing number of studies support the beneficial role of HMG-CoA reductase inhibitors, not only in the treatment of atherosclerosis but also for other vascular pathological conditions such as hypertension. Interestingly, the combined use of statins with other cardiovascular drugs could represent an important advance in the treatment of patients at risk of CHD, leading both to a reduction of the dosage and better protection, due to different, possibly synergistic, effects.

References

1. Castelli WP, Anderson K. A population at risk: prevalence of high cholesterol levels in hypertensive patients of the Framingham Study. Am J Med 1986; 80 (suppl 2A): 23–32.

2. Ferro CJ, Webb DJ. Endothelial dysfunction and hypertension. Drugs 1997; 53: 30–41.

3. Marin J, Rodriguez-Martinez MA. Role of vascular nitric oxide in physiological and pathological conditions. Pharmacol Ther 1997 75; 111–134.

4. Takemoto M, Egashira K, Usui M et al. Important role of tissue angiotensin-converting enzyme activity in the pathogenesis of coronary vascular and myocardial structural changes induced by long-term blockade of nitric oxide synthesis in the rat. J Clin Invest 1997; 99: 278–287.

5. Ichichi T, Usui M, Kato M et al. Downregulation of angiotensin II type 1 receptor gene transcription by nitric oxide. Hypertension 1998; 31: 342–348.

6. O'Keefe JH, Wetzel M, Moe RR et al. Should an angiotensin-converting enzyme inhibitor be a standard therapy for patients with atherosclerotic disease? J Am Coll Cardiol 2001; 37: 1–8.

7. Bank AJ, Wilson RF, Kubo SH et al. Direct effect of smooth muscle relaxation and contraction on in vivo human brachial artery elastic properties. Circ Res 1995; 77: 1008–1016.

8. Raij L. Hypertension and cardiovascular risk factors – role of the angiotensin II–nitric oxide interaction. Hypertension 2001; 37: 767–773.

9. Hornig B, Landmesser U, Kohler C et al. Comparative effect of ACE inhibition and angiotensin II type 1 receptor antagonism on bioavailability of nitric oxide in patients with coronary artery disease: role of superoxide dismutase. Circulation 2001; 103: 799–805.

10. Faggiotto A, Paoletti R. Statins and blockers of the renin-angiotensin system – vascular protection beyond their primary mode of action. Hypertension 1999; 34: 987–996.

11. Hoogwerf BJ, Young JB. The HOPE study. Ramipril lowered cardiovascular risk, but vitamin E did not. Cleve Clin J Med 2000; 67: 287–293.

12. Lonn E, Yusuf S, Dzavik V et al. For SECURE Investigators. Effects of ramipril and vitamin E on atherosclerosis: the study to evaluate carotid ultrasound changes in patients treated with ramipril and vitamin E. Circulation 2001; 103: 919–925.

13. Teo KK, Burton JR, Buller CE et al. Long-term effects of cholesterol

lowering and angiotensin-converting enzyme inhibition on coronary atherosclerosis: the simvastatin/enalapril coronary atherosclerosis trial (SCAT). Circulation 2000; 102: 1748–1754.

14. MacMahon S, Sharpe N, Gamble G *et al*. Randomized, placebo-controlled trial of the angiotensin-converting enzyme inhibitor, ramipril, in patients with coronary or other occlusive arterial disease. PART-2 collaborative research group. Prevention of atherosclerosis with ramipril. J Am Coll Cardiol 2000; 36: 438–443.

15. Zanchetti A, Crepaldi G, Bond MG *et al*. Systolic and pulse blood pressures (but not diastolic blood pressure and serum cholesterol) are associated with alterations in carotid intima-media thickness in the moderately hypercholesterolemic hypertensive patients of the Plaque Hypertension Lipid Lowering Italian Study (PHYLLIS). J Hypertens 2001; 19: 79–88.

16. Horiuchi M, Akishita M, Dzau VJ. Recent progress in angiotensin type 2 receptor research in the cardiovascular system. Hypertension 1999; 33: 613–621.

17. Bennai F, Morsing P, Paliege A *et al*. Normalizing the effect of nitric oxide synthase by low-dose AT1 antagonism parallels improved vascular morphology in hypertensive rats. J Am Soc Nephrol 1999; 10 (suppl 11): 104–115.

18. Bernini F, Corsini A, Raiteri M *et al*. Effects of lacidipine on experimental models of atherosclerosis. J Hypertens 1993; 11 (suppl 3): S61–S66.

19. Taddei S, Virdis A, Ghiandolni L *et al*. Restoration of nitric oxide availability after calcium antagonist treatment in essential hypertension. J Hypertens 2001; 37: 943–948.

20. Oparil S, Bakir SE. Calcium antag-onists in cardiovascular disease. Clinical evidence from morbidity and mortality trials. Drugs 2000; 59: 25–37.

21. Pitt B, Byington RP, Furberg CD *et al*. Effect of amlodipine on the progression of atherosclerosis and the occurrence of clinical events. PREVENT Investigators. Circulation 2000; 102: 1503–1510.

22. Zanchetti A, Rosei EA, Dal Palu C *et al*. The verapamil in hypertension and atherosclerosis study (VHAS): results of long-term randomized treatment with either verapamil or chlortalidone on carotid intima-media thickness. J Hypertens 1998; 16: 1667–1676.

23. Zanchetti A, Bond MG, Hennig M *et al*. Risk factors associated with alterations in carotid intima-media thickness in hypertension: baseline data from the European Lacidipine Study on atherosclerosis. J Hypertens 1998; 16: 949–961.

24. Matsuda Y, Akita H, Terashima M *et al*. Carvedilol improves endothelium-dependent dilation in patients with coronary artery disease. Am Heart J 2000; 140: 753–759.

25. Brehm BR, Wolf SC, Bertsh D *et al*. Effects of nebivolol on proliferation and apoptosis of human coronary artery smooth muscle and endothelial cells. Cardiovasc Res 2001; 430: 439.

26. Brehm B, Bertsh D, von Fallois J, Wolf SC. β-blockers of the third generation inhibit endothelin-1 liberation, mRNA production and proliferation of human coronary smooth muscle and endothelial cells. J Cardiovasc Pharmacol 2000; 36 (suppl): S401–S403.

27. Broeders MAV, Doevendans PA, Bekkers BCAM *et al*. Nebivolol: a third generation β-blocker that augments vascular nitric oxide release – endothelial β2-adrenergic receptor-mediated nitric oxide

production. Circulation 2000; 102: 677–684.

28. The Capricorn Investigators. Effect of carvedilol on outcome after myocardial infarction in patients with left-ventricular dysfunction: the Capricorn randomised trial. Lancet 2001; 357: 1385–1390.

29. Laufs U, La Fata V, Plutzky J, Liao JK. Upregulation of nitric oxide synthase by HMG-CoA reductase inhibitors. Circulation 1998; 97: 1129–1135.

30. Endres M. Laufs U, Huang Z et al. Stroke protection by 3-hydroxy-3-methylglutaryl (HMG)-CoA reductase inhibitors mediated by endothelial nitric oxide synthase. Proc Nat Acad Sci USA 1998; 95: 8880–8885.

31. Mueck AO, Seeger H, Lippet TH. Fluvastatin reduces endothelin secretion of cultured human umbilical vein endothelial cells. Eur J Clin Pharmacol 1999; 55: 625–626.

32. Wagner AH, Koehler T, Rueckschloss U et al. Improvement of nitric oxide-dependent vasodilation by HMG-CoA reductase inhibitors through attenuation of superoxide anion formation. Arterioscl Thromb Vasc Biol 2000; 20: 61–69.

33. Cooke JP, Tsao PS. Cytoprotective effects of NO. Circulation 1993; 88: 2451–2455.

34. Corsini A, Pazzucconi F, Pfister P et al. Inhibitor of proliferation of arterial smooth muscle cells by fluvastatin. Lancet 1996; 348: 1584.

35. Mitani H, Bandoh T, Ishikawa J et al. Inhibitory effect of fluvastatin, a new HMG-CoA reductase inhibitor, on the increase in vascular ACE activity in cholesterol-fed rabbits. Br J Pharmacol 1996; 119: 1269–1275.

36. Downs JR, Clearfield M, Weis S et al. Primary prevention of acute coronary events with lovastatin in men and women with average cholesterol levels: results of ACAPS/TexCAPS. JAMA 1998; 279: 1615–1622.

37. Borghi C, Prandin MG, Costa VF et al. Use of statins and blood pressure control in treated hypertensive patients with hypercholesterolemia. J Cardiovasc Pharmacol 2000; 35: 549–555.

38. Tonolo G, Melis MG, Formato M et al. Additive effects of simvastatin beyond its effect on LDL cholesterol in hypertensive type 2 diabetic patients. Eur J Clin Invest 2000; 30: 980–987.

39. Marchesi S, Lupattelli G, Siepi D et al. Short-term atorvastatin treatment improves endothelial function in hypercholesterolemic women. J Cardiovasc Pharmacol 2000; 36: 617–621.

40. Nazzaro P, Manzari M, Merlo M et al. Distinct and combined vascular effects of ACE blockade and HMG-CoA reductase inhibition in hypertensive subjects. Hypertension 1999; 33: 719–725.

41. Sposito AC, Mansur AP, Coelho OR et al. Additional reduction in blood pressure after cholesterol-lowering treatment by statins (lovastatin or pravastatin) in hypercholesterolemic patients using angiotensin-converting enzyme inhibitors (enalapril or lisinopril). Am J Cardiol 1999; 83: 1497–1499.

Index